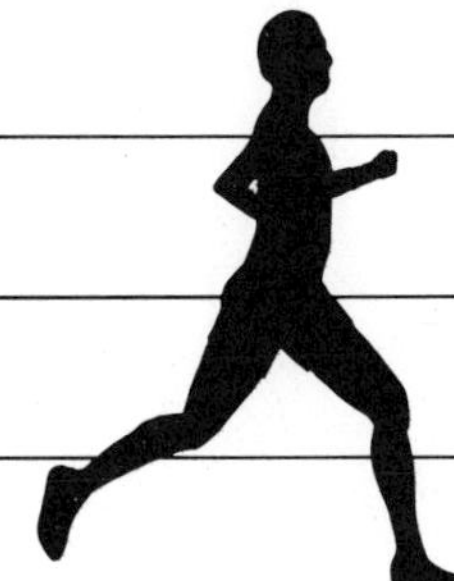

RUNNING FOR LIFELONG FITNESS

A Scientific and Personal Guide

Robert N. Girandola, Ph.D., Ed.D

University of Southern California, Los Angeles

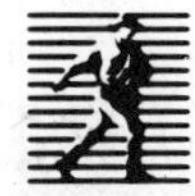

PRENTICE HALL

Englewood Cliffs, New Jersey

Library of Congress Cataloging-in-Publication Data

Girandola, Robert N.
Running for lifelong fitness.

Bibliography: p.
Includes index.
1. Running. 2. Physical fitness. I. Title.
GV1061.G57 1987 613.7′1 87–12422
ISBN 0–13–783937–5 [pbk]
ISBN 0–13–783945–6

Editorial/production supervision and
interior design: *Laura L. Cleveland*
Cover design: *Ben Santora*
Manufacturing buyer: *Margaret Rizzi*

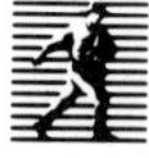

A division of Simon & Schuster
Englewood Cliffs, New Jersey 07632

Printed in the United States of America

10 9 8 7 6 5 4 3 2 1

ISBN 0-13-783945-6 01
ISBN 0-13-783937-5 01 PBK

Prentice-Hall International (UK) Limited, *London*
Prentice-Hall of Australia Pty. Limited, *Sydney*
Prentice-Hall Canada Inc., *Toronto*
Prentice-Hall Hispanoamericana, S.A., *Mexico*
Prentice-Hall of India Private Limited, *New Delhi*
Prentice-Hall of Japan, Inc., *Tokyo*
Simon & Schuster Asia Pte. Ltd., *Singapore*
Editora Prentice-Hall do Brasil, Ltda., *Rio de Janeiro*

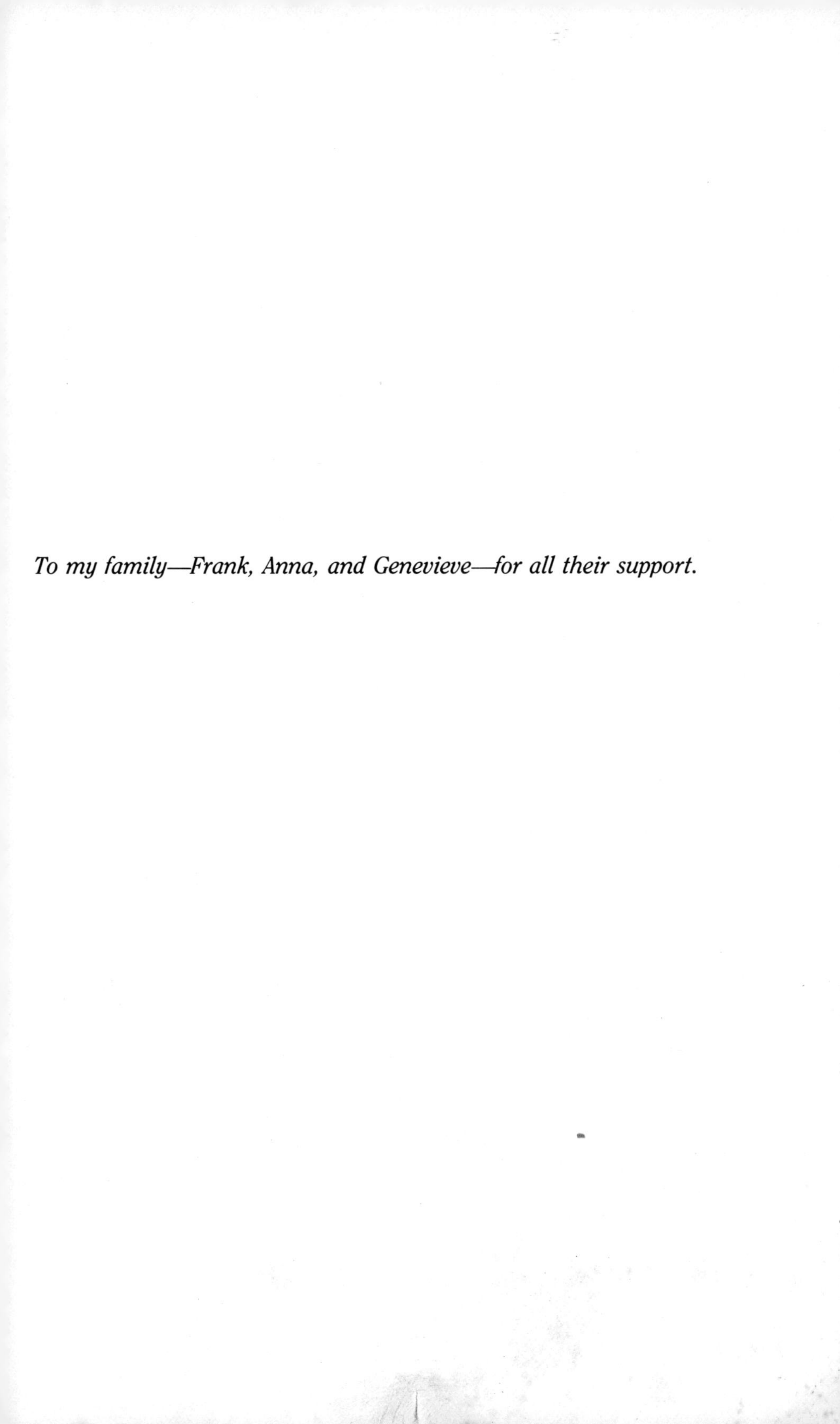

To my family—Frank, Anna, and Genevieve—for all their support.

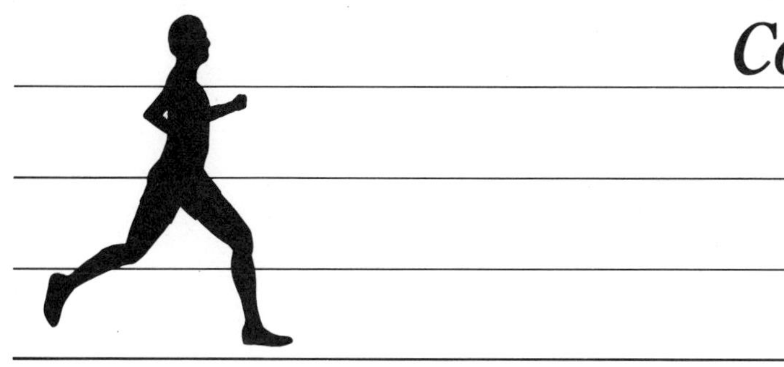

Contents

PREFACE *ix*

CHAPTER 1 Introduction

Recreation and Exercise, 1
Advantages of Running or Jogging, 2
The Popularity of Running, 3
Achievement in Running, 4
Summary, 5

CHAPTER 2 Introduction to the Physiology of Running

Biochemistry of Muscle Contraction, 7
Estimating Exercise Heart Rate, 9
Muscle Fiber Characteristics, 10
Cardiovascular Response to Exercise, 11
Running and Heart Disease, 12
Monitoring Heart Rate, 13
Respiratory Response to Exercise, 16
Metabolic Adjustments to Exercise, 17
Anaërobic Threshold, 19

Running Economy, 19
Summary, 22
Review, 23

CHAPTER 3 Psychological and Sociological Effects of Running

Runners' High, 25
Skill in Sports, 26
Psychological Benefits, 26
Summary, 28
Review, 28

CHAPTER 4 Guidelines for Setting Up a Running Program

Selection of Proper Shoes and Clothing, 29
Keeping Time, 35
Initial Training Intensity: Speed, Distance, and Frequency, 36
Training for the Marathon, 37
The Older Runner, 39
Detraining, 40
Conditioning for Running, 40
Prior Medical Examinations, 41
Summary, 42
Review, 42

CHAPTER 5 The Biomechanics of Running

Walking and Running Defined, 45
Ground Reaction Force, 46
Running Style and Form, 48
Summary, 60
Review, 60

CHAPTER 6 Injuries and Other Problems Associated with Running

Orthopedic Problems, 63
Tendonitis and Strains, 65
Shinsplints, 67
Chondromalacia, 68
Susceptibility to Injury, 68
Miscellaneous Problems, 70
Special Concerns for Young Runners, 71
Obtaining Care, 72
Dealing with Injury, 73
Summary, 73
Review, 74

CHAPTER 7 Nutritional Guidelines for the Runner

Concepts of Caloric Balance, 75
Diet and Exercise, 76
Body Composition, 79
Fundamentals of a Sound Diet, 82
What and When to Eat or Drink Before Running, 89
Summary, 90
Review, 90

CHAPTER 8 Influence of Environmental Conditions on Running

Heat, 93
Cold, 97
Altitude, 98
Air Pollution, 99
Summary, 100
Review, 100

CHAPTER 9 Stretching and Warm-Up

Stretching and Flexibility, 103
Static and Dynamic Stretching, 103
Warm-Up and Warm-Down, 104
Stretching: A Practical Approach, 105
Summary, 110
Review, 111

APPENDIX Personal Running Log 113

GLOSSARY 117

REFERENCES 125

SELECTED READINGS 129

INDEX 131

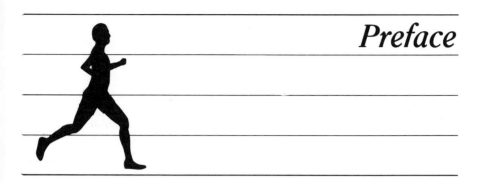

Preface

The opportunity to write a book on running was a stimulant as well as a challenge. There are so many books dealing with this topic on the market that, initially, I felt that another text could not make an additional significant contribution. However, as I evaluated several of the available running books, I realized that many important details were missing. Several books emphasized running methodology (i.e., how to run) but neglected physiological concepts. Other books discussed physiological adjustments to running but mentioned nothing about biomechanical principles. What was needed was a book for runners, and potential runners, that would explain scientific concepts, as well as methodology, in a form that was easy to read and yet did not suffer from a reduction in accuracy.

I have been an avid distance runner for the past 15 years and have completed more than 10 marathons during that time span; thus, I have experienced both the satisfactions and the pain of distance running. Having done research in the field of exercise physiology, I can discuss the benefits of running from a subjective point of view, as well as from the objective view of the scientist. I have attempted to discuss many of the practical concepts of running, as well as the beneficial and some of the detrimental effects. I have endeavored to write this text in a style that is understandable to someone without a scientific background. However, I have not sacrificed the scientific method for a simplification of writing style. For the most part, the information in the book is founded on scientific studies that can be located in reputable scientific journals, several of which I have cited. I have found that material based on personal opinion is often contrary to the scientific literature and tends to become a means of capitalizing on one's popularity at that point in time. It would be presumptuous to imply that there are no good books on running available. As a matter of fact, several have been listed in the bibliography. However, you should use good judgment in selecting the most appropriate book for your needs.

The text begins with a chapter on the popularity of running and lists some of the recent world records in distance events. Chapters 2 and 3 deal with the physiology and psychology of running. I have included some of the benefits to be derived from long-distance running, both from the standpoint of the mind as well as the body. Chapter 4 is a comprehensive discussion on how to select proper running shoes and clothing; it also covers the principles you should keep in mind when first starting a jogging or running program.

Chapter 5 deals with the biomechanics of running. Proper and improper running mechanics are discussed, as well as the problems a runner may encounter from using poor form. This is an area that is sorely lacking in most running texts on the market. Some of the more common injuries associated with long-distance running are covered in Chapter 6. I discuss causes, prevention, and treatment. A chapter on weight control and nutrition follows. Many individuals begin a running program primarily to lose weight and I cover the concepts involved. Chapter 8 discusses various environmental factors, such as heat, cold, and air pollution, that may be important to the runner. The final chapter, which includes a great many illustrations, discusses the proper methods of stretching and warm-up. The techniques discussed here are important in helping to prevent injuries that may arise as a result of continuous running.

I hope this book will answer many of the questions asked by serious joggers and runners, as well as stimulate interest in potential runners and motivate them to join this increasingly popular sport.

Acknowledgment

I would like to express my appreciation to Mario Pace for his expertise in photography in putting together the illustrations. In addition, I would like to thank Frank Jobe, M.D. (Centinela Hospital, Inglewood, California) for his assistance in obtaining photographic examples of a stress fracture and the knee joint. I would also like to thank the subjects (Julie Rollow and Quentin Sims) who patiently posed for all the photographs.

CHAPTER 1
Introduction

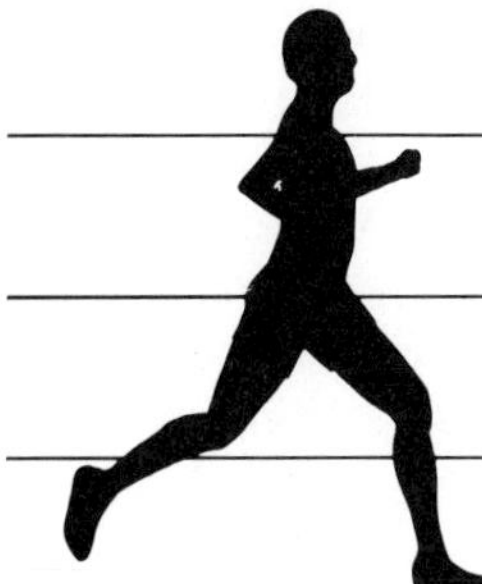

In 1979 a Gallup Poll conducted in the United States indicated that 46 percent of all Americans exercise regularly. This can be compared to a value of 47 percent in 1977; however, it shows a distinct upswing since 1961 when a poll indicated that only 24 percent of the population exercised regularly. In the poll, people were asked to list which activities they had participated in one or more times within the last twelve months. Swimming was listed by 37 percent of all respondents, bicycling was next at 27 percent, and bowling was third at 24 percent. It was also found that 12 percent of the population jogged, compared to 11 percent in 1977.

It is interesting to note the large percentage of individuals engaged in recreational activities at this point in time as compared to twenty years ago. If Gallup polls had been available in the early 1900s, there may have been an even smaller number of individuals engaged in recreational activities. What are some of the reasons for the much larger audience participation in activities over the past fifty to sixty years? Certainly some of the reasons can be attributed to the interest level of the participants, skill level, facilities (swimming pools, bowling alleys, etc.) and advertising. Another important reason can be attributed to the shortened work day, and even the shortened week (three to four days rather than five to six), which allows more time for other activities.

Recreation and Exercise

One of the major reasons for the large interest in recreational activities (especially the more vigorous ones such as aerobics, swimming, bicycling, and running) is the total lack of movement most people experience during their typical work day. Whereas farmers and blue-collar workers predominated forty to fifty years ago, today the majority of America's work force is made up of white-collar professionals. In addition, the improvement in mechanization has made many blue-collar jobs merely supervisory. Farming has become mechanized, as have construction, industry, etc. The basic implication for the changes in job descriptions over the past fifty years is that the average worker today expends a considerably smaller number of *calories* (food energy) during his or her employment compared with the worker five or six decades ago. Adding to this increasing *sedentarianism*, the mechanized world "saves" us the calories of walking up stairs (elevators), walking (cars and motorcycles), and even slicing food (electric knives). Of course, it would be an omission not to mention the development of television, which has made spectators out of millions of individuals.

The net result of this change in life style over this time period is important to consider. Many Americans have developed into fat, lazy individuals. It is estimated that more than 40 percent of Americans are obese and overweight. People become overweight as a direct result of eating more calories than they expend as energy. Therefore, it may be implied that Americans, on the average, eat more food than they really need. However, is this really a problem of too much food intake? It has been estimated that the average American male consumes about 3400 calories per day. Interestingly, the average West German and Dane consumes about the same number of calories (Caliendo, 1979) and yet there are far fewer obese individuals in these countries. For the most part, obesity is not a serious problem in most European countries and it is believed that this is due to a much more active life style.

Advantages of Running or Jogging

With all of the various recreational activities available, why should you take up running? Many people might prefer playing basketball, football, or racquetball to running three or four miles around a track. It would not be accurate to say that running is the best exercise or that everyone should run, but there are some major advantages to participating in this activity. First, several scientific research studies have shown that *endurance-type exercise* (as compared to sprinting-type, high-intensity exercises) is primarily responsible for improvements in cardiovascular functioning and decreasing body fat (Astrand, Guharay, & Wahran, 1968; Holloszy, 1973). Most individuals believe that any activity (such as football, baseball, basketball, volleyball, etc.) is classified as endurance training. In reality, the classical endurance-type activities are running, swimming, cycling, and cross-country skiing.

Another major advantage that running has over many of the recreational sports is that you are the only participant necessary to obtaining a good workout.

Playing a game of basketball requires a minimum of four to six people and a full-court game requires as many as ten players. A game of football may require as many as twenty-two individuals. Often these sports are played only once or twice a week and do not serve the requirement for daily activity. The final advantage to running is that very little equipment and no special facilities are needed. Even in an activity as simple and popular as swimming, you must have access to a body of water. You can run in an urban setting or on mountain trails; all you need is a pair of running shoes.

The Popularity of Running

How popular are running and jogging as activities? Perhaps the individual who has had the greatest positive influence on running in the United States is Dr. Kenneth Cooper. In the late 1960s, Dr. Cooper, then a colonel in the U.S. Air Force, published the now famous book entitled, *Aerobics*. Not only did this book popularize running but it helped to disseminate a great deal of the scientific information about the benefits of aerobic training. Dr. Cooper was able to simplify a great deal of the scientific terms so that the lay public was able to understand and comply with the guidelines.

In 1975, a National Health Interview survey estimated that there were four million white male runners in the United States between the ages of 20 and 59 years. It is estimated that the number of women runners has been increasing rapidly over the last several years but men runners still outnumber women runners two to one. Another recent survey (1984) conducted at the Disease Control Center in Atlanta estimated that there are presently about 12 million Americans who list running as a major activity. Nearly 40 percent of the surveyed runners ran three to five times per week, and 44 percent ran 20 to 39 minutes per session. Organized road races and marathons have also been on the increase. Figure 1 shows the increase in the number of marathon races from 1968 to 1976. The upward trend has continued through the eighties.

Ten kilometer road races (6.2 miles) appear to be the most popular and there appears to be at least one every week in certain areas of the country. In 1980 in California there were 503 races with 190,000 finishers. Some races have become happenings in a city or community, as has occurred in New York, Boston, and San Francisco. The New York City marathon, a relative newcomer, drew 17,000 official entrants in 1985. It is estimated that another 5,000 to 10,000 were "unofficial" entrants. The annual "Bay-to-Breakers" 7.6 mile run in San Francisco had an estimated 80,000 runners at the starting line in 1985. The popularity of road races is certainly not limited to the United States as can be seen by the 20,000 participants in the "Sun to Surf" 14 kilometer road race held in Australia. One thing is certain, you will not lack for company when running in these road races.

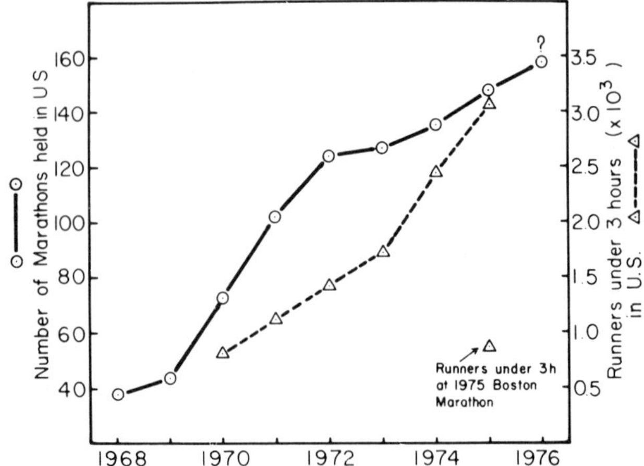

FIGURE 1. The number of marathon races held in the United States (○———○) *from 1968 to 1976 and the number of runners finishing the race within 3 hours* (△------△). (From M. B. Maron and S. M. Horvath, "The Marathon: A History and Review of the Literature," *Medicine and Science in Sports* 10 (Summer 1978), 137–150. Copyright © 1978 by the American College of Sports Medicine. Reprinted with permission.)

Achievement in Running

Most individuals who get involved with running as an activity become extremely time conscious. That is, they are usually interested in running faster as their training progresses. It is also quite natural to compare one's running times to those of the elite runners, who have set world records in their events. The marathon, which covers 26 miles, 385 yards, has long been considered the ultimate challenge for distance runners. Although world records are kept for this event it should be mentioned that marathon courses vary widely in terms of geographical terrain and climatic conditions. World records are usually set on flat courses where there are a minimum of hills and under acceptable weather conditions (cool temperatures). At present, the men's marathon record is held by Carlos Lopes of Portugal who ran 2 hours, 7 minutes, and 11 seconds at Rotterdam, The Netherlands. It is interesting to note that the average pace was approximately 4 minutes, 50 seconds per mile. The women's marathon record was set by Ingrid Kristiansen of Norway who ran 2 hours, 21 minutes, and 6 seconds in April 1985 in London, England.

Of all the distance races for which records are kept, the mile has received the greatest publicity. Roger Bannister of Great Britain was the first to break the 4 minute barrier in 1954, being timed in 3:59.4. Since then, the time for running the mile has been decreasing steadily. Jim Ryan of the United States ran the mile in 3:51.1 in 1967 and held the record for eight years before John Walker of New Zealand ran 3:49.4 in 1975.

Today, records are kept for the metric mile (1500 meters) and 6 percent longer American mile (the mile is 5,281 feet, whereas the metric mile is 4,950 feet). Most international competitions are performed over the metric distances. The men's mile record is presently held by Steve Cram of Englånd who covered the distance in 3:46.31. The metric mile record was set by Said Aouita of Morocco, who ran 3:29.45. The women's records for the mile and 1500 meters are currently held by Mary Slaney of the United States (4:16.71) and Tatyana Kazankina of the Soviet Union (3:52.5), respectively.

Summary

The increased popularity of running has paralleled the increase in time spent for recreational activities in the United States over the past fifty years. The major impetus for the running movement, however, came about in the late 1960s with the publication of Dr. Ken Cooper's book, *Aerobics.*

Records for long-distance running events appear to be broken every few months. Most people who become involved in distance running are interested in comparing their times to the record for that event or distance. However, for the recreational runner, records should be kept only as a source of motivation.

CHAPTER 2

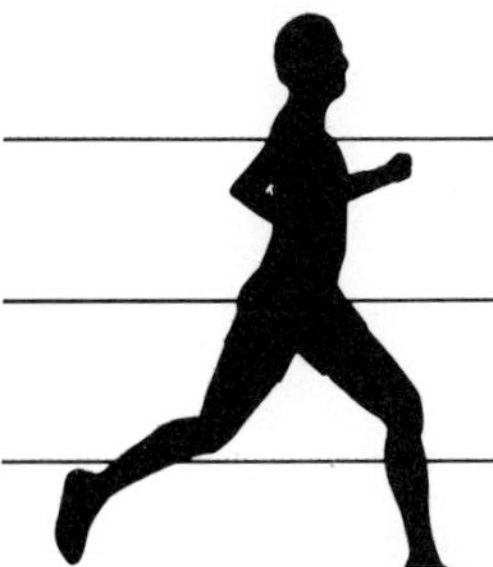

Introduction to the Physiology of Running

Biochemistry of Muscle Contraction

When you begin to exercise, your muscles begin to consume large amounts of fuel. The harder you work, the more fuel is consumed, which can be likened to the increased fuel consumption of an automobile as you depress the accelerator. The fuel that the muscle cells require for contraction is called ATP (*adenosine triphosphate*), a high-energy substrate found in all cells in very small amounts. The amount of ATP stored in muscle cells is relatively small which means that other sources of energy must be converted to this substance. The process, involving complex biochemical pathways, is called *cellular energetics*. It is somewhat similar in concept to the process of refining crude oil from the ground into the more readily usable gasoline.

Formation of ATP—Glycolysis

The categories of foods that the cells can break down to ATP are carbohydrates, fats, and proteins. Under most circumstances, protein is rarely used as a fuel but it is extremely important for normal tissue resynthesis. When carbohydrates are used for fuel, they enter the process called *glycolysis* where glucose (simple sugar) is acted on by ten different enzymes and is converted to pyruvate. During this process, two ATPs have been formed. Another name for glycolysis is the *anaerobic cycle*. The term *anaerobic* literally means without oxygen. However, a better explanation of the system would be that it is predominant during high-intensity exercise. *Lactic acid*, which is believed to be responsible for muscle fatigue, is a byproduct of glycolysis, especially during high-intensity exercise such as sprinting. Figure 2 gives a graphic representation of this process.

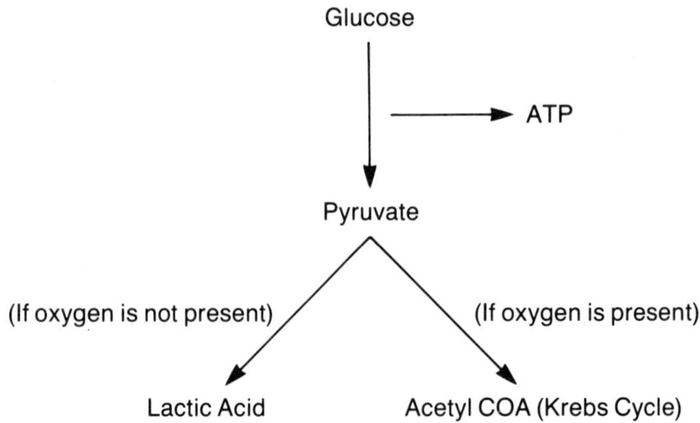

FIGURE 2. A simplified schematic of glycolytic (anaerobic) energy production. Lactic acid is produced when oxygen supply becomes deficient.

Energy Yield

Following glycolysis, the sequences of cellular energetics are called the *Krebs cycle* and the *cytochrome system*. In these processes, the pyruvate formed in glycolysis is completely broken down to CO_2, H_2O, and thirty-four ATPs. The energy yield (ATP) from aerobic processes is much greater than from anaerobic ones. In addition, it is only under aerobic conditions that fats (and proteins) can be broken down for fuel. However, since fats have a much greater caloric density than carbohydrates, they yield many more molecules of ATP per molecule of substrate utilized. Taking a typical free fatty acid (stearic acid), a total of 147 ATPs are formed. Figure 3 displays the basics of the aerobic system.

Importance of Oxygen

During exercise, it is desirable to obtain the energy for muscle contraction from aerobic processes. There is much greater efficiency and fat can also be utilized as a fuel. In order for aerobic energy production to occur, oxygen must be supplied to the muscle cell and this is, in turn, carried out by the blood in the vascular system. Oxygen supply can be increased by increasing the rate at which blood is flowing through the vascular system *or* by increasing the carrying capacity of the blood. In addition, there have to be enough capillaries perfusing the muscle tissue in order for the blood to be delivered. The key to all this is that, in order for aerobic metabolism to produce energy, oxygen must be supplied and utilized effectively, otherwise glycolysis tends to predominate with the concomitant production of lactic acid.

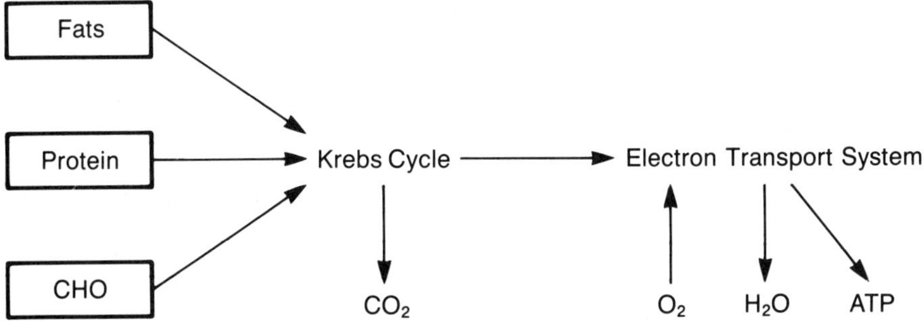

FIGURE 3. A simplified schematic of aerobic energy production. This system can function normally as long as the circulatory system supplies sufficient amounts of oxygen.

How do you ensure that sufficient blood and oxygen are being supplied to the muscle cells, specifically the legs? Assuming that you are healthy and possess an adequate amount of blood and hemoglobin, the answer deals with exercise intensity. During physical work (i.e., exercise), the major controlling variable that determines the proportion of aerobic or anaerobic metabolism is the intensity of that work, relative to the individuals' maximal capacity.

Heart Rate

In general, running at less than 70 percent of your maximum capacity ensures that the majority of energy is supplied by the aerobic system. For most individuals, running above 70 percent of their maximum involves a substantial anaerobic component. The simplest method you can use to determine running intensity is to monitor your heart rate during exercise. Maximal heart rate (HR) is usually taken as 220 minus age. Thus a 20-year-old has a maximal HR of approximately 200 beats per minute. If he or she were to jog for three miles and the measured HR during the run was 120 beats per minute it could be assumed that this individual was exercising at 60 percent of his or her maximal.

Estimating Exercise Heart Rate

To calculate the percentage of your exercise capacity:

1. Subtract your age from 220.
2. Divide that number into the measured heart rate per minute.

TABLE 1. Maximal Heart Rate Percentages for Various Ages

	Age (years)							
Measured HR	16	20	24	28	32	38	40	46
120	58	60	61	62	63	65	66	68
140	68	70	71	72	74	76	77	79
160	78	80	81	83	85	87	89	90
180	88	90	91	93	95	98	100	102
200	98	100	102	104	—	—	—	—

3. Multiply by 100 percent.
4. The answer is the percentage of maximal heart rate.

For example, if you are 20 years old and your measured heart beat rate was 120 beats per minute, the maximal heart rate percentage would be 60 percent:

$$220 - 20 = 200; \qquad \frac{120}{220} = 0.60 \times 100\% = 60\%$$

Generally, running at less than 70 percent of maximal capacity involves aerobic energy production, while exceeding 70 percent involves anaerobic energy production (see Table 1).

Muscle Fiber Characteristics

Many years ago, biochemical research on animal tissue revealed that the fibers making up one complete muscle (e.g., *gastrocnemius* and *soleus*) were not all *homogenous*. Early experiments classified muscle fibers as being either red or white. The red fibers appeared to have more hemoglobin (and myoglobin) among other properties. Today, muscle fibers are commonly differentiated by mechanical properties, such as being fast twitch (FT) or slow twitch (ST). Fast twitch fibers have greater anaerobic capabilities, contract very rapidly, are able to exert a great deal of tension or force, but fatigue rapidly. Slow twitch fibers, on the other hand, contract slowly, do not exert much tension, but are highly fatigue-resistant. Biochemically, these fibers have many *mitochondria*, which are the structures that contain the enzymes for aerobic energy production.

ST-FT Ratios

It is certainly obvious that ST muscle fibers are better suited for endurance work, that is, sustained contractions at low tension levels, and FT muscle fibers are more suited for speed, strength, and power activities. In the past fifteen years, the muscle biopsy technique (surgical removal and analysis of muscle tissue) has allowed a great deal of research to be completed on human subjects. The usual biopsy areas are the quadriceps (front of the upper leg) and gastrocnemius and soleus (calf). In the average, untrained male, there is about a 60–40 ratio, ST to FT muscle fiber composition (actually, 58 percent ST), in the gastrocnemius. Middle-distance runners were found to have 62 percent ST fibers in this muscle. Marathon and other long-distance runners had 79 percent ST fibers (Costill, Fink, & Pollock, 1976).

Why would there be such a large difference between average men and marathoners? Did physical training make the difference? More likely these differences are due to genetic endowment. So far, research has failed to show any major changes in fiber composition as a result of a training program. This means that if a person is born with a large percentage of FT muscle fibers in his or her legs it would be unlikely that he or she could ever become an *elite* distance runner. However, it does not imply that someone could not become a long-distance runner; the distinction being made is between the average runner and the elite, international-caliber performer. It is apparent that genetic endowment plays a major role in determining future athletes.

How can you determine your muscle fiber composition? At present, it is unlikely that the average person can have this evaluation done. It is considered a surgical procedure that is not without some risks and, therefore, the technique is usually performed only as part of a scientific research study. Perhaps in the near future more sophisticated instrumentation will create a less traumatic technique for the subject.

Cardiovascular Response to Exercise

The cardiovascular system is comprised of the heart (pump), vessels (arteries, veins, and capillaries), and blood (red and white cells and plasma). The function of this system is to supply blood (with oxygen) to the various tissues of the body and also to help in temperature regulation. There are approximately 5 liters (quarts) of blood in the vascular system and, under normal resting conditions, that volume makes one complete circuit in one minute. In other words, normal resting cardiac output (blood flow) is about 5 liters per minute. When you begin to exercise, that value increases substantially. The average unconditioned male may achieve a cardiac output of about 16 liters per minute during maximal exercise. This can be compared to some extremely well-conditioned endurance athletes (runners and cross-country skiers) who have achieved cardiac outputs of close to 40 liters per minute!

It is apparent that there is a major cardiovascular adjustment to exercise. Although there is still some argument about this in the scientific community, it is believed that the cardiovascular system is the major limiting factor to endurance performance. This means that an individual who has a very large cardiac output should be able to outperform an individual who has an average cardiac output, in terms of distance-type activities. It has been shown that endurance-trained runners have stronger and more functional hearts. More specifically, it was found that the thickness of the walls was greater, they had larger ventricular muscle mass, higher diastolic (filling) volume, and improved ventricular function. It should be comforting to note that when you run for distance (at least a mile and preferably longer) you are helping to develop your cardiovascular system.

Running and Heart Disease

Some scientists and clinicians have stated that long-distance running is the best protection against heart disease. Indeed, many people run (and do other exercises) in the hope that they will not suffer heart attacks. Yet you often hear about supposedly well-conditioned individuals who have died of heart attacks, some at a relatively young age. The recent and untimely death of Jim Fixx, who suffered a heart attack while jogging, left many would-be runners in a state of apprehensive confusion. One reason that many individuals take up jogging as an activity is that they may decrease the risk of heart disease. You can only imagine what they may be thinking after reading about cardiovascular accidents occurring during jogging, especially in someone in such "apparent" good health as Jim Fixx.

If an individual has an advanced case of atherosclerosis it is likely that he or she may suffer from a mild or severe heart attack if subjected to a bout of heavy physical exercise. There have been many documented cases of sedentary middle-aged men suffering a heart attack during the exertion of shoveling snow on a winter day. It is important that everyone understand the risk factors of heart disease as well as the diagnostic procedures available to identify the problems. In the case of Jim Fixx, apparently there was relatively severe atherosclerosis present in the coronary blood vessels. Post-mortem publicity revealed that Mr. Fixx had a family history of heart disease and he himself was an overweight, heavy smoker until he undertook his running program. It was also discovered that he did not obtain medical advice regarding his cardiovascular health. It may very well be that Mr. Fixx was able to prolong his life, somewhat, by undertaking the running program he adopted.

Some of the major risk factors in cardiovascular disease include obesity, high serum cholesterol, hypertension, stress, diabetes, smoking, and a sedentary life style. It would be foolish to expect that running several miles a day would prevent heart disease in all individuals, unless the other risk factors (and family history) in each person could be ascertained. It is certainly accepted that the risk of heart disease in long-distance runners is lower than in the general population. However, it is not known, with absolute certainty, whether the running conferred this lower risk or whether genetics played the major role.

It is known that runners possess stronger hearts with more muscular walls and more efficient energy usage. This is caused by a much slower rate of contraction (heart rate) with concomitant increase in blood ejection per beat (stroke volume). There is speculation that endurance exercise causes an increase in coronary collateral circulation. That is, there are a greater number of blood vessels (or total cross-sectional area of the vessels) that supply the heart with blood. Although studies on animals have proven controversial (both pro and con), there have been no studies on humans to date that have successfully substantiated this hypothesis.

Several recent studies found that long-distance runners have a greater proportion of high-density lipoproteins (HDL) in their blood when compared to similar-aged populations of sedentary males. Evidence indicates that individuals with higher levels of HDLs in their blood have a lower risk of heart disease (Hartung, Foreyt, & Mitchell, 1980; Adner & Castelli, 1980). It is also accepted that running (as well as other endurance-type activities) positively affects some of the other heart disease risk factors. Running has been found to decrease the percentage of body fat (obesity), decrease blood pressure in some cases (hypertension), and help decrease stress. Individuals who take up a running program (or any other physical activity), especially for the first time or after a long sedentary interval, should be aware of the risk factor for heart disease, as well as their family histories related to this disease. A sound medical examination should be encouraged prior to engaging in any vigorous physical activity.

Monitoring Heart Rate

Most individuals who decide to get involved in a running program are extremely interested in knowing how their body adapts to physical stress. The single physiological variable that is both informative and simple to measure is the heart rate. In the laboratory, the heart rate is usually monitored by the use of chest electrodes and an apparatus called the *electrocardiogram* (EKG). In the field, you can monitor your heart rate using relatively inexpensive monitors. Those that attach to the chest and measure the electrical activity of the heart tend to be the most accurate and reliable. Examples of this can be seen in Figures 4 and 5.

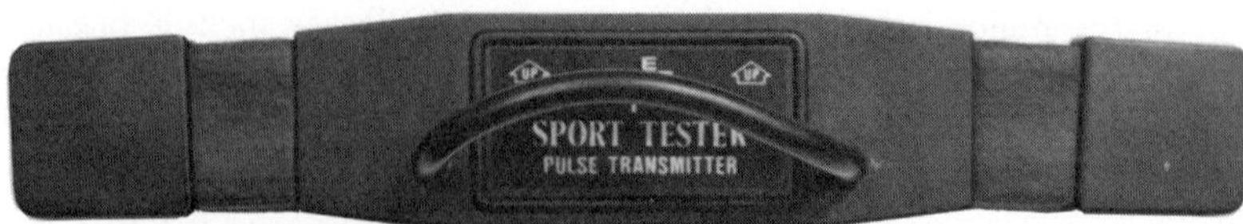

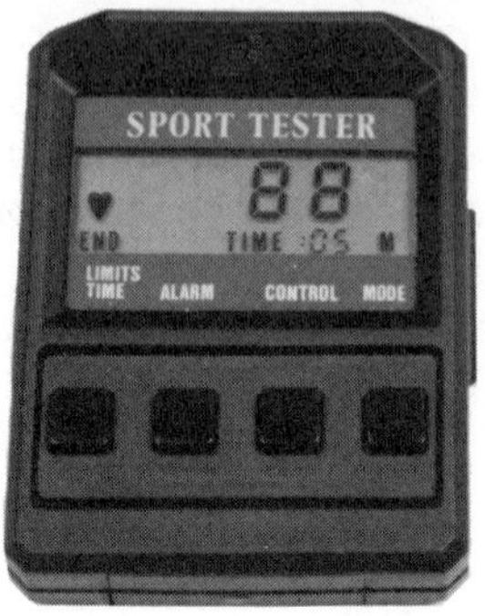

FIGURE 4. A typical, commercially available heart rate monitor.

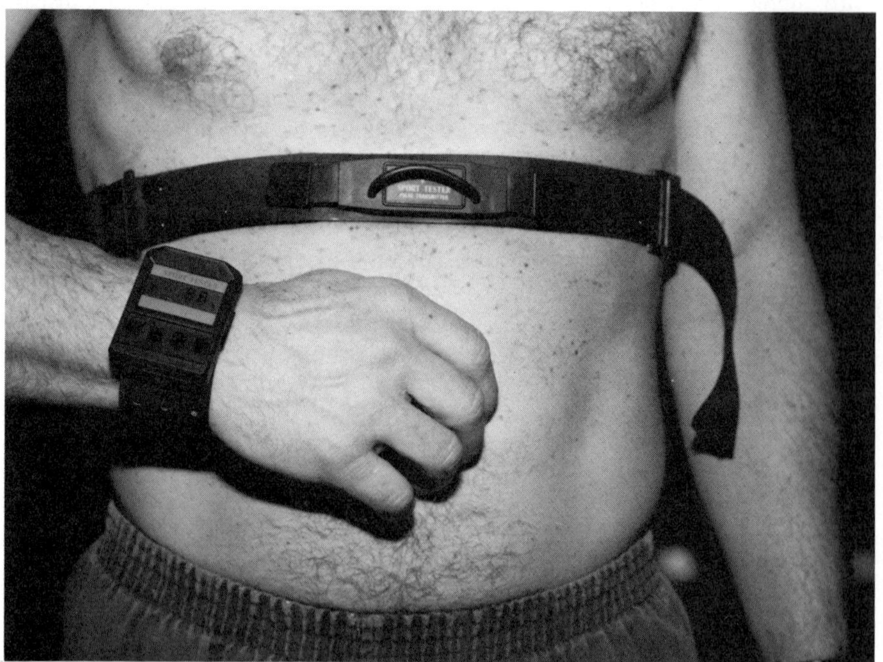

FIGURE 5. The heart rate monitor is attached to the runner's chest. The digital receiver is worn like a watch.

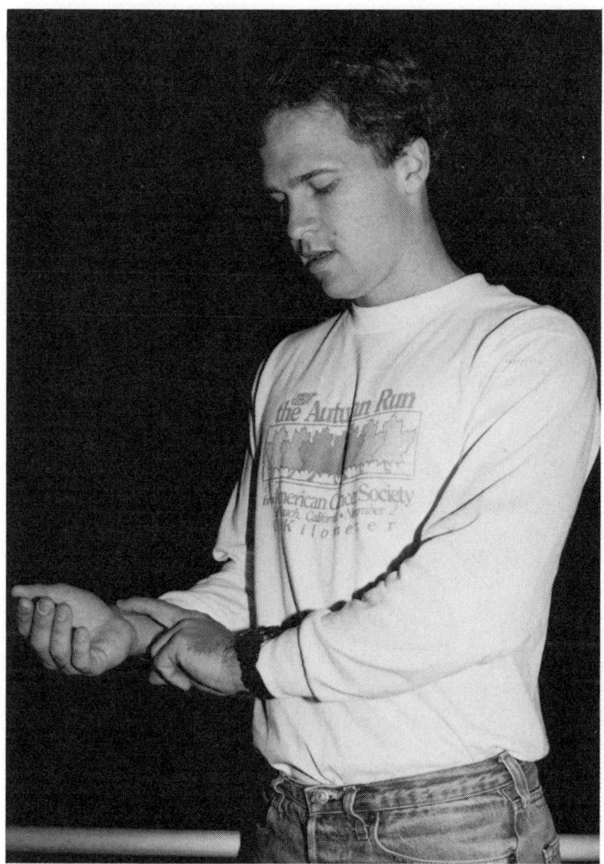

FIGURE 6. The subject palpates his radial pulse (wrist, on thumb side) to monitor his heart rate.

You can also monitor pulse rate (the pulsations of the blood that are related to the contractions of the heart) manually using only your fingers and a stop watch. This can be done by palpating (feeling with the fingers) one of the superficial arteries, the most common sites being the brachial and carotid areas (see Figures 6 and 7).

The usual procedure is to use the middle and index fingers of one hand and press gently over the area, feeling for the pulsations created by the blood. Count the pulses for 10 or 15 seconds and convert to a one-minute score (multiply by 6 or 4). Keeping track of resting HR can be valuable because the decrease that occurs over time is one of the most reliable indicators of an endurance training response. In addition, measuring HR during running is an excellent indicator of the relative stress or intensity of the exercise.

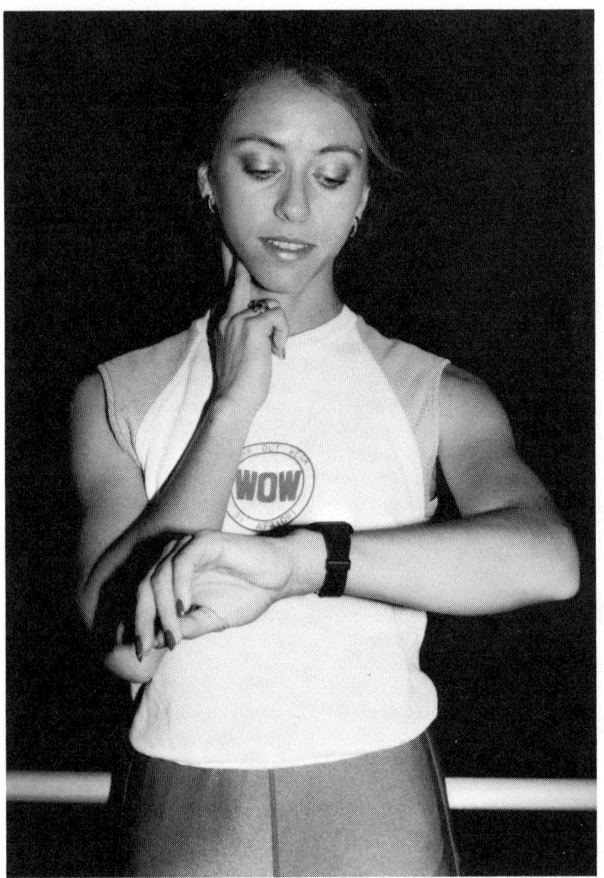

FIGURE 7. The subject palpates her carotid pulse (on neck, below jaw) to monitor her heart rate.

Respiratory Response to Exercise

The respiratory system is comprised of the mouth, nose, trachea, bronchi (small tubes connecting the trachea to alveoli), and alveoli (tiny air sacs). Its major function is to ventilate air and diffuse oxygen into the blood and CO_2 out of the blood. At rest an individual probably ventilates about 10 to 15 liters of air per minute. During maximal exercise a strong, healthy individual may exceed 200 liters per minute. Compared to sedentary individuals, well-conditioned athletes can usually ventilate more air during maximal exercise. This is due to the fact that the trained person has stronger muscles in the chest, abdomen, and shoulders, which aid in ventilation. However, despite the apparent effects of training, it should not be construed that ventilation is a limiting factor in exercise in normal subjects.

Wind

Many runners who become fatigued almost invariably feel that it is their lungs that "gave out." The statements most often used are, "My wind gave out" or "I ran out of air." Subjectively, most people feel that the fatigue originates in the respiratory system. In spite of these feelings, research has conclusively shown that in the normal, healthy person, the lungs are not the limiting factor in exercise. Even after an individual reaches his or her subjective maximum, there is still a substantial pulmonary reserve. In other words, the individual fatigues before he or she reaches maximal ventilatory capacity. However, it should be emphasized that this rule holds true for healthy lungs only. When people smoke or have asthma or some other pulmonary dysfunction, pulmonary function may very well be a limiting factor in exercise capacity.

Breathing Pain

Almost everyone who has run has, at some point, experienced sharp pains in the sides of the abdomen and chest. This pain, often referred to as a *stitch,* is more frequent in poorly trained individuals. Many people believe it is due to drinking water or other cold fluids prior to exercising. Fluid ingestion is rarely the cause of this disturbance. Although it has not been proven conclusively, most researchers believe the pain is caused by fatigue of the diaphragm or the accessory respiratory muscles, usually the intercostals (located between the ribs). It is not considered a serious problem, except that the pain may cause the individual to stop running. As training progresses, these pains should decrease in both frequency and severity.

Metabolic Adjustments to Exercise

Perhaps the single most important measure that can be used to evaluate endurance athletes is *maximal oxygen consumption* (VO_2 max). It is also referred to as aerobic power. Although it is basically a measure obtained in the laboratory, it is much less difficult to obtain than cardiac output. Studies have shown that VO_2 max is the most important variable in determining success in running distances up to 6 miles.

VO_2 max is usually expressed as the amount of oxygen consumed per kilogram of body weight (i.e., ml O_2/kg/min). An average college-age male may have a VO_2 max of 45 ml O_2 and a similar-aged female, 38 ml O_2. Some elite male distance runners and cross-country skiers have been measured at around 80 ml O_2/kg/min. These values are due to extremely high cardiac outputs and a high proportion of slow twitch muscle fibers, which were discussed previously.

As you get into better physical condition by running, the VO_2 max can be expected to increase, and you will find it easier to run faster and longer distances. Both men and women should expect to improve at about the same rate (more about this in Chapter 4), although women will average about 15 percent less than men at almost all training levels.

Figure 8 demonstrates the method of obtaining maximal oxygen consump-

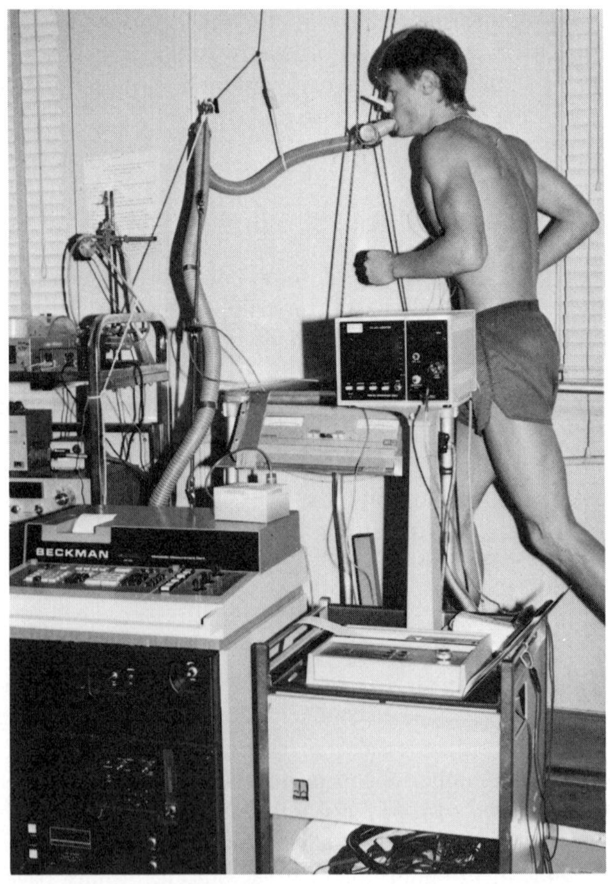

FIGURE 8. Measuring maximal oxygen consumption in the laboratory involves the use of a treadmill (or bicycle) and sophisticated gas analysis equipment. The subject runs until he cannot maintain the pace of the treadmill.

tion in the laboratory. The subject runs on the treadmill to his or her subjective maximum while breathing into a two-way breathing valve. Expired air is continually analyzed for the percentage of oxygen and carbon dioxide. The procedure, although somewhat costly if done in a commercial fitness facility, is extremely informative and can provide some valuable information regarding adaptations that occur during a period of training.

Anaerobic Threshold

Another important variable that has recently received a great deal of attention is the concept of the anaerobic threshold (AT). The AT, usually expressed as a percentage of your maximum, is the exercise level where anaerobic energy production (and lactic acid) increase dramatically. In running long distances (6 miles and greater), it is important to run at a pace that is below your AT. If you run above the AT then the likelihood of your finishing the race (especially one as long as a marathon) is not very good since the lactic acid produced will probably cause fatigue.

Although there is not a great deal of information about this area, it appears that the average person has an anaerobic threshold of approximately 60 percent of maximum. Studies on some elite distance runners indicate their ATs to be around 85 to 90 percent. This could explain how these athletes are able to run so fast (5 minutes per mile and faster) for so long (26 miles). As with many other physiological variables, (e.g., cardiac output, muscle fiber composition, etc.), the AT is most probably determined by hereditary factors. However, studies indicate that training improves the value somewhat (Davis, Frank, Whipp, & Wasserman, 1979; Costill and associates, 1971).

Running Economy

Running economy can be defined as the amount of energy required to run at a given pace, for a given distance, for an individual of a certain weight. Often, the term *efficiency* is substituted for running economy. *Efficiency*, however, is defined as the amount of energy required to do a certain amount of work. From an absolute definition, the differences in efficiency between two individuals doing the same task (e.g., running at the same pace) is very small. What actually transpires while performing seemingly similar tasks is that some individuals are quite skilled and movement patterns are finely tuned. Even in an event such as running, which appears to be quite simple in terms of motor coordination, there appear to be large differences between individuals in terms of gait patterns and overall body movements. If you have a great deal of extraneous movement while running, such as up and down or side to side, the actual amount of work you do is greater than in someone who has minimal movement. Therefore, if you do more work per stride run, the amount of energy required per stride increases. The sum total is that the smoother and more effective the movement patterns while running, the more economical you will become. Running economy is extremely important in long-distance running since it helps save "fuel" which might otherwise become depleted.

Studies show that, even in relatively well-trained runners, there are substantial differences in terms of running economy. Marathon runners were found to be about 5 to 10 percent more economical than middle-distance runners (see Figure 9).

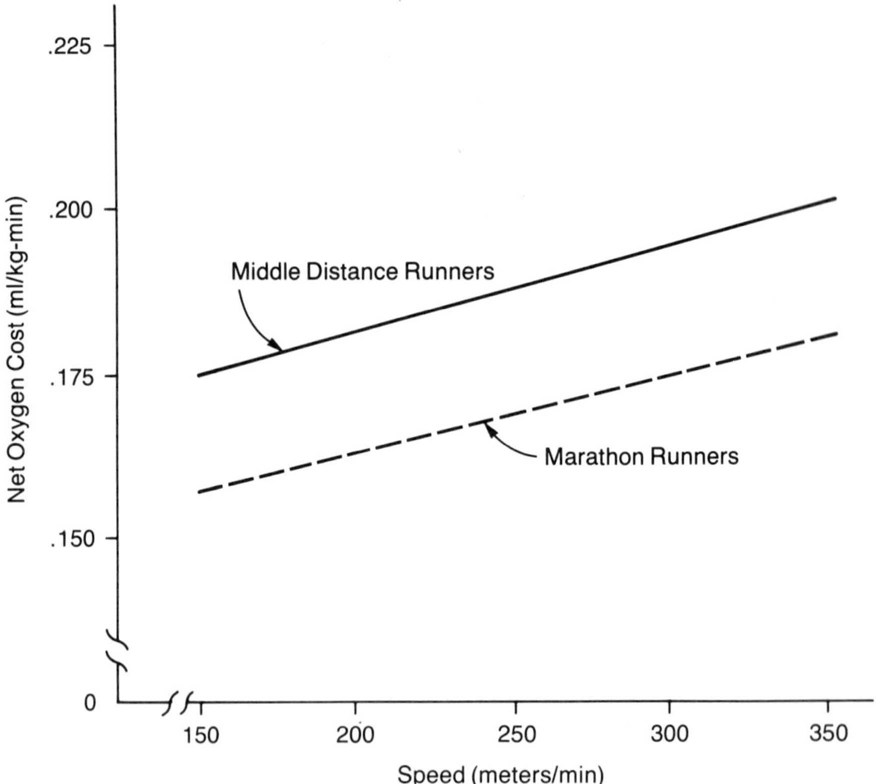

FIGURE 9. A comparison of net oxygen cost (energy) of level running for middle-distance (———) and marathon (- - -) runners. (Adapted with permission from D. L. Costill, "Physiology of Marathon Running," *Journal of the American Medical Association* 221(9) (August 1972): 1024–1029. Copyright © 1972 by the American Medical Association.)

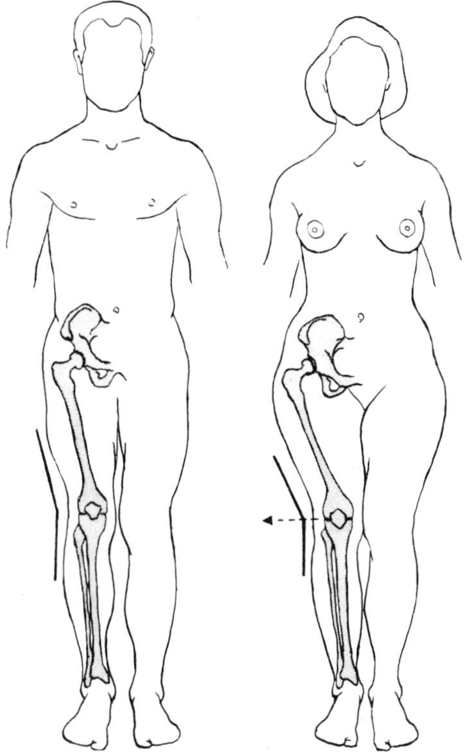

FIGURE 10. The broader pelvis of the female on the right results in a greater angle of the femur. Weight-bearing and angle of push-off may not be as efficient. (From D. O'Donoghue, *Treatment of Injuries to Athletes*, 3rd ed. (Philadelphia PA: W. B. Saunders, 1976), p. 613. Copyright © 1976 by W. B. Saunders Co. Reprinted with permission.)

Economy, Sex, and Age

Some people believe that during running, women are less economical than men because of structural differences in the hips (see Figure 10). As you can clearly see from the diagram, the angle of the large, upper leg bone (femur) in women is directed more inward (creating a slight angle between outer pelvis and knee joint). This is in contrast to the almost vertical (180 degrees) plane of the male femur. Anatomically, this is due to the wider flare of the female pelvis (hip) that begins to develop at puberty in response to the increased secretion of female sex hormones (estrogen). It has been speculated that this slightly inward tilt of the femur results in greater energy expenditure and, possibly, more frequent knee injuries. However, the data of several scientific studies failed to substantiate either of these speculations. It should also be noted that many lean females do not exhibit the wider pelvis and angled femur of their heavier counterparts. Perhaps some of the structural anomaly may be due to menstrual irregularities resulting from low body fat and/or intense training. This will be discussed more fully in Chapter 7.

Research shows that children are less economical than adults during running. Again the speculation is that children have not yet developed good running form at early ages (9 to 15 years). Whenever you run, it is important to maintain good form and keep extraneous movements to a minimum.

Running Economy and Wind

Running into a strong wind or up a steep hill drastically increases the amount of effort you have to put forth, compared to running on level ground or with no wind. While running, about 5 to 8 percent of the energy spent is needed to overcome air resistance. As the wind against you increases, so does the energy expenditure. Thinner people have an advantage here because their body structure offers less resistance to the wind.

Running Economy and Hills

Running up hill increases energy expenditure tremendously. Studies show that running up a 6 percent incline requires about 35 percent more energy than running at the same pace on level ground. In these studies, when the subjects ran *down* the 6 percent grade their energy output was 24 percent less than during level running. This means that you use more energy running up and down hills than running on level ground. In addition, there appear to be marked differences in economy in runners during hill running. This may explain why some individuals seem to relish running hills while others simply abhor them.

Summary

The physiological and biochemical adjustments to exercise, or more specifically, running were described. The production of ATP (fuel) at the cellular level, with the concomitant need for oxygen and blood delivery, was discussed. A simplified method of monitoring pulse rate and exercise intensity was evaluated. The relationship of heart disease to running was discussed, with an emphasis on understanding some of the risk factors of the disease, as well as the preventive effects of jogging. In addition, the effects of running on pulmonary function and metabolic rate were covered.

Review

1. ATP is produced as a result of the metabolic breakdown of fat, protein, or CHO. The metabolic breakdown occurs in the muscle cell as a result of specific enzymatic pathways.
2. The enzymatic pathways are designated as being anaerobic (without oxygen) or aerobic (with oxygen). The aerobic pathway is more effective and is the main one used in endurance-type exercise.
3. The cardiovascular system supplies blood to the muscle cell and is highly developed in an endurance-trained athlete, such as a runner.
4. While there is no direct evidence that running, as a training program, prevents heart disease, there is a great deal of evidence that it may reduce some of the risks of the disease.
5. Maximal oxygen consumption is an important measure because it can be used to evaluate relative success in long-distance running.
6. The anaerobic threshold and running economy are additional measures that can be used to evaluate a runner's potential success.
7. There are differences in running economy between children and adults. Although anatomical differences exist between males and females, these have not resulted in lower economy for females.

CHAPTER 3

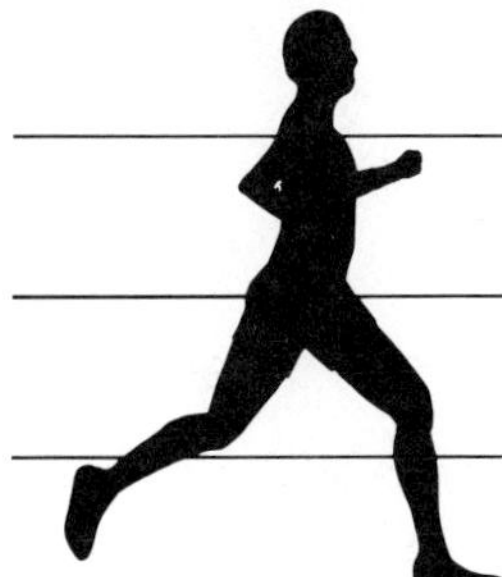

Psychological and Sociological Effects of Running

While it is apparent that the majority of individuals who undertake a running program do so because of the physiological benefits, many runners choose the sport because of the psychological and sociological benefits they receive. Personal satisfaction and contacts with other runners serve as the major motivation for many men and women.

Runners' High

Much has been said about the addicting quality of running. Some runners talk about reaching a "runner's high" during a long workout. This "high" has been described by some as a "higher level of thinking," a "clarity of mind," a "transcendental state of being," or simply as "euphoria." Whatever this feeling might be, it is apparent that running in itself creates a state of well-being in some individuals, whether it occurs during or after the run.

There has been some speculation, based on research in this area, that the "runner's high" may actually be attributed to the presence of morphine-like drugs called *endorphins* in the central nervous system. Some scientists have gone so far as to postulate that these endorphins may be related to individual differences in pain threshold. As an individual trains longer, more of this drug may be secreted by the central nervous system. This might explain why better trained or conditioned individuals are more able to tolerate pain in running. Furthermore, it suggests that different individuals can reach differing states of the "runner's high" (Stein & Belluzzi, 1978). It should be emphasized, however, that while many runners claim that they are able to get a "high" from their workout, many others claim no such benefits from the sport. Perhaps this is an individual phenomenon or perhaps it is in the individual's state of mind.

Skill in Sports

Many individuals have been frustrated as children and later as adults while attempting to participate in many of the skilled sports such as baseball, football, tennis, volleyball, and swimming. Most of these sports require a great deal of practice time in order to become proficient. The poorly skilled or uncoordinated individual may have had to spend many painful hours watching from the sidelines or being the last player to be picked in a game. While running does require some motor coordination, it really cannot be classified as a skilled activity. It offers almost anyone the satisfaction of active competition. Today, there are many highly proficient runners with a great deal of public notoriety who were probably unskilled athletes in school games. The psychological benefit of being able to accomplish something in sport, such as winning a 10-kilometer race, or finishing a marathon, is unquestioned.

Psychological Benefits

From a personality standpoint, it has been documented in several studies that in many individuals a program of regular exercise is extremely beneficial in reducing both anxiety and depression. The evidence in a recent study at Purdue University indicates that depression is the major component of emotional stability that varies between active and sedentary groups. Utilizing the Minnesota Multiphasic Personality Inventory, a group of 40 to 60-year-old joggers was compared to a similar-aged sedentary control group; it was found that the joggers displayed little evidence of depression.

Several earlier studies attempted to identify personality differences between runners and nonrunners. In general, it was revealed that runners had a tendency to be more creative and imaginative, more trusting and accepting, and less anxious or depressed. A high degree of mature or "adult" characteristics were found to prevail among many of the tested runners. Greater emotional stability, persistence, and conscientiousness were among the common traits observed (Hammer & Wilmore, 1973; Buccola & Stone, 1975; Hartung & Farge, 1977). Although these traits appear to be desirable, the studies also showed that runners displayed some undesirable characteristics. Runners often display aggressive behavior and tend to be driven and goal-oriented, sometimes to the point of foolishness. A recent article even likened distance running to anorexia nervosa, which is a psychological disorder where the patient, because of a distorted body image, literally starves himself or herself to death. Anorexia patients are driven individuals who strive for a skeleton-like appearance. The implications are that runners tend to drive themselves in the same manner.

Running provides an attractive exercise modality for the middle-aged and older adult, women, and even children. Marathon running has long been associated with individual success in the late twenties. Whereas most track and field records are often set by teenagers and those in their early twenties, long-distance running records are often set by those in their late twenties and even in their early thirties. Witness the recent success of Carlos Lopes of Portugal, who won the men's marathon in the 1984 Los Angeles Olympics at the ripe "old" age of thirty-seven. Many men and women in their sixth and seventh decade of life participate on a regular basis in long-distance running. These individuals (aside from the physiological benefits) benefit from their ability to train for and compete in rigorous physical challenges. To a certain degree, the training may act as a "psychological rejuvination" for them.

Although women have been competing at an increasing level in competitive sports of all kinds over the last ten years, there has never been anything as dramatic as the increase in the number of competitive women runners. The 1984 Olympics saw the introduction of the first women's marathon in Olympic competition. The psychological benefits women receive include greater confidence in themselves, greater independence, and a stronger self-concept. Although many women feel that they cannot compete with men in sports on an equal basis, they may in reality discover that they can run faster and further than many men. Women now possess the knowledge that they can undergo the same stress that remained formerly in the domain of the male world. Many women runners do not see themselves as the "weaker" sex. The rise of women in the business, academic, and political worlds can, in many ways, be attributed to the increasing awareness of their own physical as well as mental capabilities.

As in the case with women, there has been an increase in the number of juvenile participants in road races. There is little, if any, evidence dealing with the psychological effects of running on children. However, the ability to persevere at a task, to accomplish the extremely difficult, and to compete with adults appears to have a beneficial effect on a child's personality development. There is always the danger, however, that the child may be pushed into the sport by parents and expectations may be set too high. Children should be allowed to run when they wish and, although some encouragement should be given, they should never be forced to do something because the parents feel it is best for them.

Although running is considered an individual sport, one that individuals can compete in by themselves, in reality it is far from the solitary activity that many people perceive it to be. So many people run today that you can often find running partners in any park and on any street corner. Fifteen or twenty years ago, it would have been unbelievable to find someone running down the streets of midtown Manhattan in New York City. Today you can find men and women alike who don running clothes, carry their suits in a backpack, and actually run to work. Noontime in most large cities finds a multitude of joggers using their lunch hour as a running break.

However, the real "social scene" occurs in the sponsored road races. As previously mentioned, it is not unusual for 5,000 to 10,000 individuals to be entered in a race. Although some individuals are quite competitive, the majority are usually quite sociable and you can strike up a conversation with a perfect stranger, and keep it going for a few hours, in the case of the marathon races. The encouragement that you receive from spectators during a long road race is incomparable to any other feeling in competitive sports. Even the individual who is at the back of the pack, who may be running at an incredibly slow pace, is vociforously encouraged. Running *can* be a solitary activity, but more often it becomes an activity to renew interpersonal relationships and create a social scene that helps keep most people highly motivated.

There is some scientific evidence to indicate that runners display better emotional traits, when compared to sedentary control subjects. Whether these personality traits were developed as a result of a running program, or the individuals possessed these traits before they began running, is not known. It would appear that there may be some psychological benefits that an individual would obtain from exercising on a regular basis, running being an excellent example. The older individual and women in general may obtain the greatest personality benefits. It is suggested that running be carried out under pleasant conditions and surroundings to infer the greatest pleasure. Allowing the running to become an all-consuming obsession is not advisable since there may be unwanted psychological as well as physiological repercussions.

Summary

Of what psychological benefit to an individual is a regular program of running? This is what has been discussed in this chapter. Although there is some objective evidence to substantiate certain claims, the majority of statements relating the psychological benefits of running remain subjective and anecdotal.

Review

1. The euphoria that many runners experience while out on a long run may be traced to the secretion of a morphine-like drug called *endorphin* by the central nervous system.
2. Runners display more favorable personality traits when compared to individuals in other sporting endeavors.
3. As a result of the great number of participants in road races, running has become a socially interactive sport.

CHAPTER 4
Guidelines for Setting up a Running Program

Selection of Proper Shoes and Clothing

As was stated in Chapter 1, running requires the least amount of equipment and facilities, when compared to any other competitive or recreational sport. Shorts, shirts, and a pair of running shoes are all that are necessary. For the most part, it is a relatively inexpensive participant sport. However, as with any fad that has increased in popularity, there is an advent of commercialism. Numerous sporting goods stores have cropped up selling all kinds of knickknacks for the runner. Some of these items may be important to certain individuals (such as cotton visors to keep both the sun and perspiration out of your eyes or a special pouch to keep keys or money in), but many of these gimmicks are just a means of milking the public of money. For instance, many feel it is important to be seen running in attractive warm-up suits. Some of these warm-up suits are extremely expensive and, although they may look good, they often have little functional service. However, as stated earlier, to many running is a social scene and appearance is often more important than the running itself.

Shoes

Without question, a good pair of running shoes is the most important equipment acquisition that you will make. Several years ago, purchasing a pair of running shoes was a relatively simple matter since there were only a few different types of shoes on the market. This is certainly not the case today. There are several major running shoe manufacturers (i.e., Nike, Brooks, New Balance, Adidas, among others) and each company may have as many as ten different models to choose from. Included in this list are shoes for men and women and training versus racing models. It is somewhat perplexing to make a shoe selection from such a vast array. However, the large selection also allows the experienced and knowledgeable runner to make an intelligent choice. This runner will be able to pick a shoe that meets his or her rquirements and perhaps will help solve some of the biomechanical deviations that are common to most individuals.

The following factors should be kept in mind when evaluating a pair of running shoes:

Rearfoot and forefoot impact response. As will be discussed in the biomechanics chapter, the amount of force imparted between foot and ground during running is two to three times body weight. Therefore, the running shoe should partially absorb some of the impact. With the development of newer, lightweight, shock-absorbing material, impact response of shoes has really improved over the past five years. The midsole of the shoe (see Figure 20, Chapter 5) is responsible for cushioning and it is usually made from ethylene vinyl acetate (EVA) and/or polyurethane. Many shoes are designed especially for individuals with special problems such as pronation or supination. For example, in the case of over-pronation, a multidensity midsole is used. Materials having different firmnesses are placed in specific locations, greater cushioning where the heel strikes but firmer material on the medial aspect of the shoe.

Rearfoot control. This is a measure of excessive motion at the rear of the shoe. Modern running shoes have gone a long way in helping eliminate this problem with the development of external heel counters. Basically, this structure helps hold the heel in place when it hits the ground, which is important in trying to control over-pronation.

Sole traction. This aspect of the shoe determines its ability to maintain traction with the ground. Different sole patterns have efficiencies and limitations depending on the surface you are running on. A concrete path can be slippery when wet and a sandy track can become muddy or dry out to become gravelly. Each surface characteristic affects the traction of the shoe sole and the efficiency of running performance.

Flexibility. This refers to the flexibility of the longitudinal aspect of the shoe. Holding the heel of the shoe and bending the toe section upwards indicates the degree of flex. In general, the greater the motion control the shoe offers, the stiffer the shoe. Therefore, you may have to sacrifice certain aspects or qualities of a shoe in order to obain certain other qualities.

Weight. Running shoes become lighter each year. The use of air soles and heels and EVA midsoles have allowed manufacturers to lighten modern day shoes. As a matter of fact, today's training shoes are as light as the racing shoes of a few years ago. To a certain degree, the lighter the shoe, the less motion control (stability) and impact response the shoe will possess. Although light shoes are desirable, the weight of the shoe should not be the criterion upon which you make a selection. Although a heavier shoe will increase the amount of work you do while running (but only a small amount), it also offers greater cushioning and motion control.

Training and Racing Shoes

There are basically two types of running shoes—training and racing models. The major difference between the two categories is weight and height differential from forefoot and heel. Racing shoes are usually lighter than training shoes. In a copy of *Runner's World* a few years ago, the average men's training shoe weighed 320 grams while the average racing flat was 235 grams (a difference of about 3 ounces). Most of the standard training shoes have a three-layered heel with a differential of ¾ to 1 inch between forefoot and heel. Racing shoes are essentially flat with no height difference between forefoot and heel. Unless you are involved in competitive running, racing shoes are not recommended, since there is a greater possibility of musculoskeletal injuries from long-term use.

Selection of Shoes

Modern running shoes, such as those in Figure 11, are designed to meet the demands of every type of runner, including the heavy-weight person, the person who has wide or narrow feet, and the person who has problems with motion control. Shinsplints, which were a common problem for runners years ago, have almost been eliminated as a result of the cushioning materials used today. Custom-made shoes designed to help solve individual gait problems (see Figure 12), although done occasionally, are rarely necessary.

When you are ready to purchase a pair of running shoes, you should begin by observing the shoes and looking for loose or uneven stitches or sloppy gluing, or any other defect in workmanship. Although the quality control of the major shoe manufacturers is excellent, some poor quality shoes always slip by.

The shoes should be tried on and fitted for proper sizing. Check for proper length and a reasonably roomy toe box. The toes take a beating during long-distance running and, by having a tight fit in this area, you will exacerbate the problem. Your toes should not touch the front edge of the shoe. With the shoes on, while standing, there should be one finger's width distance between the toes and the end of the shoe. The length of walking shoes is not quite as critical since the foot does not slide forward in the shoe during normal walking. However, during running, it is common for the foot to slide forward somewhat during the landing phase of the movement. If there is no space between the toes and

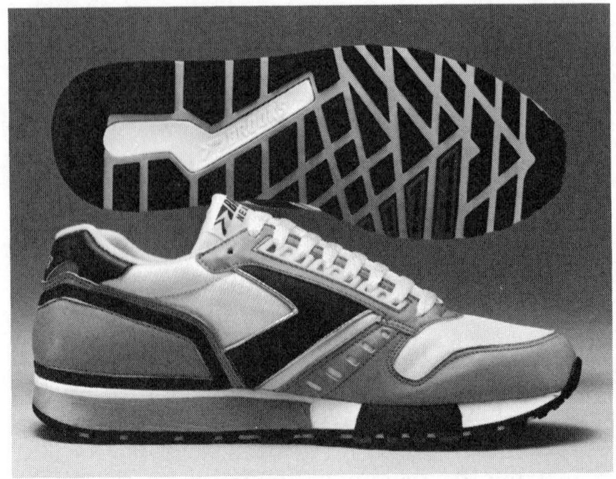

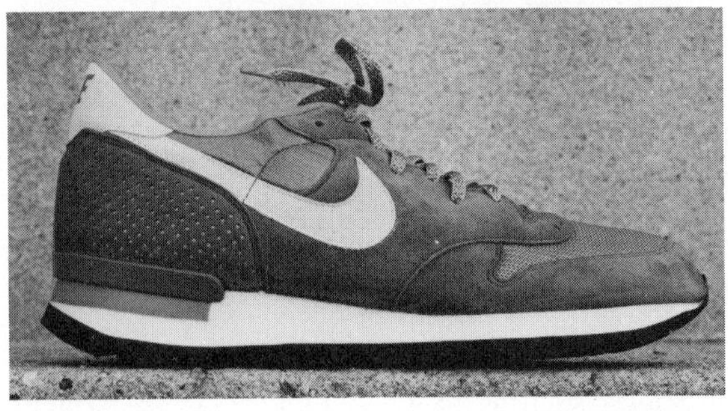

FIGURE 11. These running shoes incorporate some of the modern principles that have evolved as a result of biomechanical testing procedures. Notice the built-up heel section, including the heel counter and heel counter support. (Top photo courtesy of Brooks Shoes, Rockford, Michigan; bottom shoe is by Nike.)

the front of the shoe, the toes will be traumatized. Blisters and lost toenails are common occurrences.

The shoe should flex easily at approximately one-third of the distance from the toe. The heel counter should be tested for stiffness by squeezing it between your fingers; it should be firm and resist compression. The back and upper part of the heel counter should be soft and smooth on the inside so that it will not rub against the Achilles tendon and heel. The width of the shoes, especially near the front of the foot, is also critical. The shoes should not fit too tightly since your feet will swell somewhat during a long run. Most of the swelling is due to fluid accumulation in the foot and is quite common. Therefore, there should be some space in the shoe to allow for this.

Several manufacturers offer special shoes designed for women. However, many of these models are made from lasts (basically, the form of the shoe)

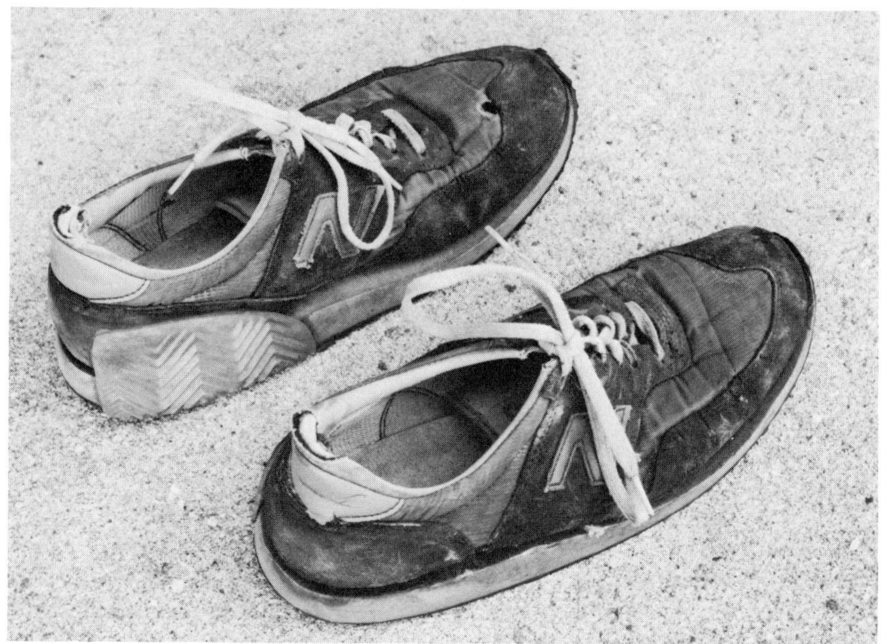

FIGURE 12. This pair of customized running shoes has certainly seen better days. The wearer of these shoes undoubtedly had a pronation problem as you can see the built-up section of the medial aspect along the posterior section of the shoe.

modified from those used for men's shoes. It appears that women's feet may be significantly different than men's. Research by Converse indicates that female runners had narrower heels, wider forefeet, and higher arches (compared to men). A study by Nike indicates that women's shoes need to be made thinner in order to give the same amount of flexibility. It is apparent that the next few years will see rapid development of running shoes made specifically for women.

Cost

The cost of running shoes has gone up considerably in the last several years. The prices usually range between $40 and $80, although there are a few exceptions. Some people will pay considerably more for a pair of street shoes but resent the large expenditure for a pair of "sneakers." Cutting costs in running shoes is probably not a very wise decision. You must understand that there has been a great deal of costly engineering conducted by each shoe company in trying to develop excellent running shoes. Engineering and research costs are usually passed on to consumers when they buy the finished product. Changes in running shoes over the past 15 years have been astounding. Only someone who has purchased running shoes over this time period could evaluate the tremendous improvement in both comfort, style, workmanship, and overall utility.

When comparing a pair of expensive street shoes to running shoes you should keep in mind that, although the street shoes may be worn for several hours each day, the average mileage covered would be comparatively small. On the other hand, most joggers put many miles a day on their running shoes. The stresses placed on the feet and lower extremities during running must be somewhat neutralized by the shoes. The importance of a good pair of running shoes cannot be minimized and, although not everyone should spend $100 for a pair, you should not buy a bargain basement brand in the hopes of saving a few dollars.

Socks

Socks serve two purposes—they help absorb some of the perspiration from the foot and they help prevent blisters that might occur as a result of abrasion between the skin and the shoe. Wool socks are best for absorbing moisture but they may be too bulky; therefore, a combination of wool and another material (cotton) is often recommended. Some individuals prefer wearing a light cotton sock or liner and then a heavier pair on top. This is personal preference. Socks should fit snugly on the foot and not bunch up or the end result will be painful blisters. Many individuals enjoy running without socks but, unless you are used to this, the end result will be some rather severe abrasions.

Outer Clothing (Shorts, Shirts, and Warm-Up Suits)

The popularity of jogging has brought forth a seemingly endless variety of clothing to be worn before, during, and after running. The rationale for wearing a warm-up suit will be discussed in Chapter 8. This is also a situation where personal preference is at issue. There is no major advantage or disadvantage, depending upon weather conditions.

Shorts and shirts should be loose-fitting and comfortable. Shorts should not bind the legs during running and shirts should preferably be tank-type (sleeveless). The use of nylon mesh material for shirts offers many advantages. Nylon is slippery and does not abrade the skin as other materials do. In addition, the small holes in the material create a more effective evaporative cooling medium.

Many people, out of preference or necessity, run in the evenings, after sunset. If running is done on a track then no special precautions need to be taken. However, if you do your running on streets with regular traffic then special attention needs to be taken with outer clothing. Several shoe manufacturers have incorporated reflective materials on the heel counter and sides of the shoe. In addition, reflective material on clothing, such as shirts, shorts, and outer sweats, should be worn. Many runners do not realize how difficult it is to observe a lone individual on the side of a road at night, especially when street lights are missing or inadequate. It is always best to be safe.

Protection from Chafing and Perspiration

One of the problems the long-distance runner faces is the chafing that occurs from clothing and the interaction from the moving limbs (i.e., inside of upper thighs and area near the armpits). Avoid clothing or other items that tend to be abrasive against the skin. (Wool is an excellent example.) Many runners carry petroleum jelly with them and apply it liberally before a long-distance event. The jelly can be applied to any area (even the feet and toes) where chafing occurs. Sometimes Band-aids can be applied, in addition to the jelly, to very sensitive areas such as the nipples. Spenco Corporation produces several items that can be helpful, including "second skin" and stick-on padding. Women may need specially constructed jogging bras in some instances.

For those who perspire a great deal, the addition of a hat or sweatband may be advantageous. Perspiration running down the face can get into the eyes and create visibility problems. An absorbent (cotton) hat or sweatband can help prevent this. In addition, a hat can protect the scalp somewhat from radiant heat when the sun is shining brightly.

Keeping Time

One final piece of equipment which is highly recommended is a digital chronograph. The cost of this item ranges from $10 to $200, depending on the manufacturer as well as the type of case and watchband material (i.e., plastic versus stainless steel or silver). A stopwatch can be used to determine your running speed over a given distance and, therefore, would be invaluable if you wish to evaluate your training program. In addition, the watch can be used to monitor heart rate (unless you have a heart rate monitor) during and after exercise and thus give information as to exercise intensity. The relatively low cost and accuracy of the present-day digital chronographs make it an almost indispensable item for the serious runner.

Initial Training Intensity: Speed, Distance, and Frequency

Perhaps the most difficult area to comment on intelligently is the initial training level. There are drawbacks to recommending a set protocol for readers of this text for two reasons. First, there are still a great deal of controversies regarding the interaction between intensity (speed), duration (distance), and frequency (number of days) of training. That is, some say intensity is most important, others say duration, and still others may vote for frequency. The second reason concerns the variability in fitness levels of those reading the text. Some individuals may be young and very fit, while others may be middle-aged and in poor physical condition. It would be very foolish to recommend one program for all individuals to adopt.

Begin Slowly

If you have never done any long-distance running, or, if it has been a long time (several years) since you have done any serious exercise, then the recommendation would be to begin *slowly*. One of the most common mistakes a novice runner can commit is to train overzealously at the beginning. This will invariably lead to muscle soreness and other injuries which may discourage you from continuing the program. What is considered slow? When you first start, try running three times per week, with one day's rest between each workout. The duration of each workout should be 30 minutes (some beginners may have to walk part of the time). The intensity or speed of the workout is the most variable component. Some beginners may be able to run at an 8-minutes per mile pace, others at a 6-minutes per mile, and still others at 12-minutes per mile. You must be able to monitor your heart rate during, or immediately following the run, in order to determine the relative intensity of the exercise. It is suggested that initial training intensity range from 60 to 70 percent of maximal. You should utilize the procedures outlined in Chapter 2.

Once you have gone beyond the novice category (after several weeks), the next step is to increase the frequency of workouts. Running five to six days per week rather than every day appears to be the choice of many runners since it allows some time for recovery. If you do not wish to be sedentary one or two days per week, then perhaps another form of exercise could be substituted. Swimming, cycling, and aerobic dancing are all excellent aerobic exercises. Running is somewhat traumatic to muscles and joints and it appears that one or two days without running may be advantageous, especially for high-mileage enthusiasts.

Increasing Intensity and Duration

After achieving the five to six day per week goal, the next step is to increase intensity and/or duration. The choice depends somewhat on your goals and schedule. For example, if your goal is to be able to run a 5-minute mile then you must train at a relatively fast pace, most of the time. In addition, if your schedule only permits 30 minutes per day for recreation then training should also be done at a faster pace. However, if your goal is to run in a marathon, then you must increase the duration of the workout, providing your schedule permits. In general, it could be said that you should train at a fast running pace if you wish to run faster competitively. If you wish to run a fast mile, then continuous, long, slow distance training will not allow you to reach your goal. Similarly, if you want to complete a 26 mile race, then running 2 to 3 miles per day, regardless of the speed, would not be very advantageous. One important point concerning pace. Studies show that the adult population does not seem to enjoy or tolerate a high-intensity training program. There appears to be a high dropout rate as well as a higher incidence of musculoskeletal injuries, when compared to a low-intensity running program.

As mentioned previously, people run to improve cardiovascular function and to reduce body weight and fat. Evidence shows that long duration and moderate intensity (60 to 70 percent of maximum) running is optimal for both. Therefore, it is recommended that you stay with this program, if these are your goals. However, it should also be kept in mind, that in order to keep improving, especially in terms of VO_2 max, you must gradually, but consistently, increase the intensity of your running program.

Interval Training

Interval training is basically very high-intensity running with short rest intervals in between. It is sometimes called *Fartlek training*. In terms of improvement in cardiovascular function, there appears to be little to choose from between interval (100 percent of maximal) and continuous (70 percent of maximal) training. If you are working on speed, you should incorporate some interval workouts in your schedule. In addition, it may be advantageous for the long-distance runner to do some interval training since it would break the monotony of long, slow distance.

Training for the Marathon

The ultimate achievement for the long-distance runner is to complete a marathon. The fact that there are so many more scheduled marathons today, as well as more participants (20,000 to 30,000 in the New York City marathon in 1985), indicates that quite a few runners are achieving this goal. Most individuals who begin a running program cannot believe that they could ever complete 26 miles, unless they had an automobile! Invariably, though, after training for several months or several years (depending on initial fitness level), many of these skeptical individuals enter and complete their first marathon. Age is not a barrier as individuals in their seventies have completed the distance, and some have done so in very respectable times.

Mileage

Although there are some differences of opinion regarding the exact training protocol for the marathon, there is one point on which there is unanimous agreement—*mileage*. In order to be able to complete 26 miles, you must train by running many miles per week. It would appear that you should be covering at least 50 miles per week prior to the race. It is usually recommended that the mileage covered Monday through Friday be kept at a moderate level, perhaps 5 to 6 miles per day. On Saturday and Sunday, when people usually have more free time, your mileage should be increased substantially to 10 to 20 miles per day. The training pace depends on your ultimate goal in the race. For example, if you would be satisfied with completing the marathon in 3½ hours, you must run the race at an 8-minutes per mile pace—and, of course, you must then train at this pace or, preferably, faster.

Fatigue

The fatigue that occurs during the course of running 26 miles (or longer) is quite different from what most novice runners are accustomed to. It is usually not the central type of fatigue, resulting in *dyspnea* (labored breathing) and general internal discomfort. Instead, the fatigue usually affects the peripheral areas, such as the legs and hips. It is generally assumed that during the very long-distance run, glycogen is depleted from the cells in the exercising muscle groups. Therefore, fuel depletion may be a major factor in the marathon, but certainly not the only limiting factor. A discussion of the methods used for increasing the level of muscle glycogen appears in Chapter 7. However, you must adapt your muscles for long-term continual contraction. The pain that accompanies the completion of a long-distance running event is a result of small tears or injury to connective tissue in the muscles and joints.

The "Wall"

Most runners have heard the term "hitting the wall" associated with the marathon. It is supposed to occur at about the 20-mile mark in the race. In reality, many runners tend to drop out of the race at this point because of the extreme pain and fatigue. Physiologists believe that the 20-mile mark is closely associated with glycogen depletion (especially in the novice runner), but there are probably other factors involved. Some well-trained individuals never suffer severe discomfort during the course of the race and, in fact, quite a few runners have completed ultra-marathons (greater than 26 miles, some as long as 100 miles). Therefore, for these runners, there is no invisible wall at 20 miles. It is recommended that, besides the high mileage training, you attempt to complete at least one long run of 20 miles (or more) prior to the marathon. This will not ensure that you will complete the race; however, your chances will be much greater. Figure 13 illustrates the improvement in running speed of winners of the Boston Marathon over the past eighty years. It is obvious that training methods must be improving.

The Older Runner

If you are an older individual, especially someone who has never exercised, you must be more cautious in your training program. Initial training intensity should be lower than that recommended for the young adult. As your training program

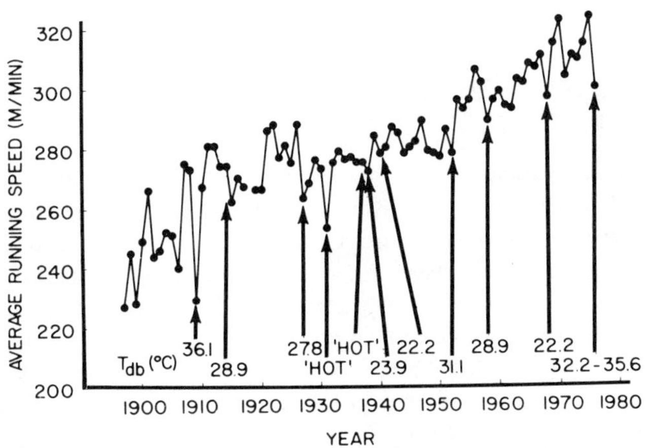

*FIGURE 13. **Average running speeds of winners of the Boston Marathon from 1897 to 1976. Race times were converted to running speeds. When data on temperature (dry bulb, °C) was available on hot days, it was included.*** (From M. B. Maron and S. M. Horvath, "The Marathon: A History and Review of the Literature," *Medicine and Science in Sports* 10 (Summer 1978), 137–150. Copyright © 1978 by the American College of Sports Medicine. Reprinted with permission.)

progresses, there is no reason to be overly concerned about extending yourself in a workout. Studies have demonstrated that even in their sixties individuals respond well to endurance training. Cardiovascular improvements are similar to those of younger subjects, but not of the same magnitude. It does take the older runner a longer period of time to get into shape, however. Evidence has shown that for every decade of age after 30, it takes about 40 percent longer for participants to progress in their training program.

Detraining

While training to get into good physical condition for running, one of the most important concepts to be kept in mind is the effect of *not* exercising. Many people mistakenly believe that if they train for a given period of time (even for several years), the effects will last forever. Unfortunately, the results of detraining are usually evident within a few short weeks. There are losses in certain contractile proteins and metabolic enzymes (in muscle cells), as well as some decrement in cardiovascular function. Studies done on subjects during enforced bed rest conditions indicate that the detraining curve closely mirrors the typical slope of the training curve. This means that you will generally lose the effects of endurance training at the same rate that you gained them.

Conditioning for Running

The long-distance runner usually has little need for specific conditioning exercises, other than running itself. This certainly does not imply that for certain individuals extra conditioning exercises (i.e., weight training and calisthenics) may not be beneficial. However, under most circumstances, typical joggers do not have to concern themselves with strengthening other parts of their bodies. Strength is not a very important component of long-distance running unless you have to do a lot of uphill work. At times, fatigue of your arms and shoulders may occur. If this happens, it may be advantageous for you to strengthen your arms and shoulders by using specific exercises.

Accessibility to free weights (barbells, dumbells) or more sophisticated Nautilus or other machine-type weights will allow you to perform the following exercises:

1. Military press
2. Bench press

3. Pull-overs
4. Curls

If weights are not available, the following calisthenic exercises are recommended:

1. Push-ups
2. Pull-ups
3. Dips (on parallel bars)

You should consult a text on weight lifting or ask for instruction from trained personnel if you are unfamiliar with these exercises.

Musculoskeletal injuries may be caused by muscle imbalance, frequently in the legs (i.e., hamstrings and quadriceps). Under these circumstances, you would benefit from specific weight-lifting exercises. Orthopedists, physical therapists, podiatrists, or chiropractors often prescribe conditioning exercises to help alleviate musculoskeletal problems.

Sit-Ups

Sit-ups are strongly recommended on a daily basis. Most individuals have very weak abdominal muscles and this often leads to back problems. Strong abdominals prevent the pelvic bone (hips) from tilting forward and downward, thus preventing excessive lower back curvature (*lordosis*). Traditional methods of strenghtening the abdominal muscles are not recommended. These include upper leg lifts with the lower leg extended and sit-ups, where the feet are anchored and the lower legs are extended. There are several methods of performing sit-ups correctly. You must make certain that your feet are not anchored down and your knees are bent at about a 90-degree angle. Sit-ups are best done before going out to run.

Prior Medical Examinations

Would it be wise to take a 4 to 5-year-old automobile, that has never been driven other than around town, on a 3,000 mile cross-country trip without first having the car completely checked out and serviced? Most experienced drivers would not do such a thing. Although the analogy is not very good, the same concept applies to the human organism. If you are relatively young (mid-twenties and younger) and in good physical condition, the necessity for a pretraining medical examination is not so pressing. However, if you are over 35 and have never been very active, it would be to your advantage to have a thorough medical examination prior to beginning a running program.

The most important aspect of the medical examination is the cardiovascular check-up. Therefore, you must visit a clinic where a cardiologist is present or available. A resting and stress electrocardiogram (EKG) is mandatory. The stress EKG is usually done on a treadmill or bicycle ergometer and essentially gives the physician information about cardiovascular pathology (disease). As valuable as the EKG is, it is not foolproof. Some physicians have even criticized the poor diagnostic capability of the EKG in relatively young, healthy individuals. However, at present, it is still one of the best noninvasive diagnostic tools available to identify any latent disease condition. Together with a chest X-ray, blood lipid analysis, blood pressure, and other aspects of the examination, the EKG should give you and the physician a valuable profile of your cardiovascular capabilities. If possible, it is recommended that the clinical facility be one where they specialize in sports medicine. The personnel, as well as the physicians, are better trained in evaluating and treating exercise-related medical problems.

Summary

This chapter is designed to help a novice or even an intermediate runner make appropriate selections for running apparel. Shoe selection is extremely important and decisions should be based on body weight, stride mechanics, running surfaces, intensity and duration of training, and, finally, comfort. In addition, guidelines for setting up a running program are presented for the short-distance enthusiast as well as the prospective marathoner. Finally, recommendations for a conditioning program and prior medical examination are presented.

Review

1. Running shoes should be evaluated for the following characteristics: rearfoot and forefoot impact response, rearfoot control, sole traction, flexibility, weight, and comfort.
2. Shoe selection should be made with regard to any gait problems you may have. Shoes must be comfortable. You should try on several pairs of shoes in your selected category, prior to making a decision.
3. Outer clothing selection should be based on comfort as well as environmental conditions you expect to run in.

4. Heart rate monitors are valuable tools for evaluating training intensity. Their cost has decreased to the point that they can be considered an important equipment purchase for the avid runner.
5. The most important concepts that must be adhered to in a training program are speed, distance, and frequency.
6. Untrained or poorly conditioned individuals must be disciplined enough to begin the training program slowly. That is, the initial intensity and duration should both be low.
7. Training for ultra-long distances, such as a marathon, requires a great deal of dedication and time.
8. Conditioning by weight-training and calisthenic exercises is recommended as an all-around program for the runner.
9. Any individual over the age of 35 years is advised to undergo a medical examination prior to undertaking any vigorous exercise program. This exam should include an exercise EKG.

CHAPTER 5
The Biomechanics of Running

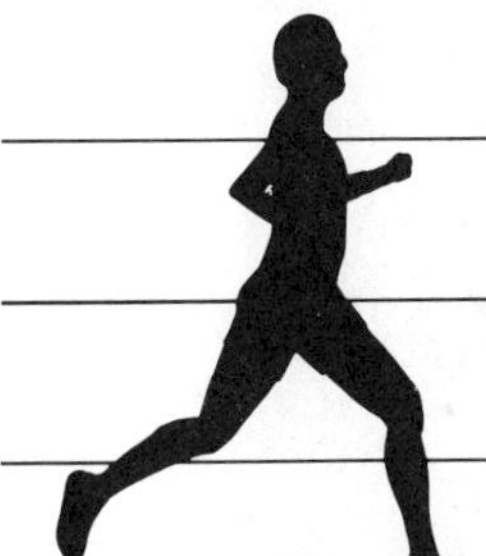

Biomechanics is the science that examines both the internal and external forces acting on a human body and the effects produced by these forces. When you apply this definition to running, an example of the internal forces is the knee joint contact force; the ground reaction (with the foot) is an example of the external forces.

Walking and Running Defined

Both walking and running are technically called *bipedal* (two-limb) locomotion. The upper trunk is balanced over the two legs which alternately swing forward. Force is imparted to the ground as each foot is pushed off. Arms are swung alternately front and back (left arm swings forward as right leg goes forward) to counterbalance the rolling action of the pelvis. Technically, running is the same as walking, but with some major differences. In walking, one foot is always in contact with the ground (see Figure 14). During walking, the stance or support phase occupies about 60 percent of the cycle (one cycle is two consecutive foot strikes of the opposing legs). As you progress to race walking and, finally, to running, this phase occupies a smaller and smaller percentage of the total cycle.

An individual walks slowly (relative to running) and, therefore, there is a relatively small force imparted to the ground from the contact foot. What this means is that there is little vertical deflection of the body during horizontal movement. On the other hand, during the running action, there is a nonsupport phase in which both feet are in the air at the same time. Figures 14, 15, and 16 illustrate the relative differences in body movement in the same subject during a walk (3 MPH), slow run (6 MPH) and fast run (9 MPH). One can see that in

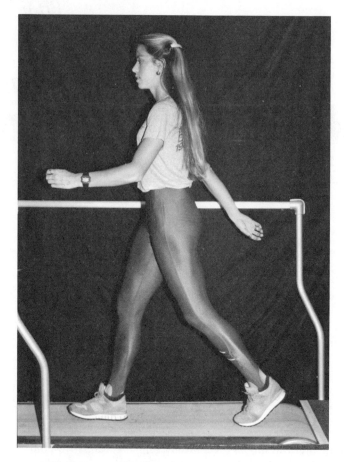

FIGURE 14. The subject is walking at a speed of about 3.5 MPH. Notice that both feet are in contact with the ground surface.

the fast run the subject appears to be several inches off the ground with both feet.

Ground Reaction Force

Since horizontal speed is greater in running, more force must be generated by the contact foot and this in turn leads to more vertical deflection. Side-to-side deflection is also characteristic of running. In running, the impact with which the foot hits the ground has been calculated to be between three to four times

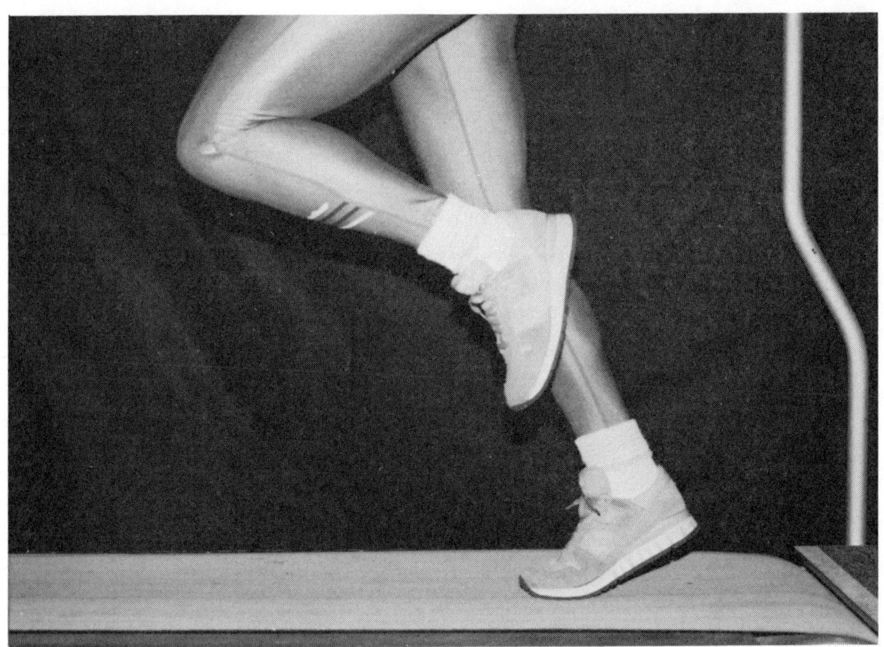

FIGURE 15. The same subject runs on the treadmill at a moderate speed. Notice that one foot is well off the running surface and the knee lift is higher than in walking.

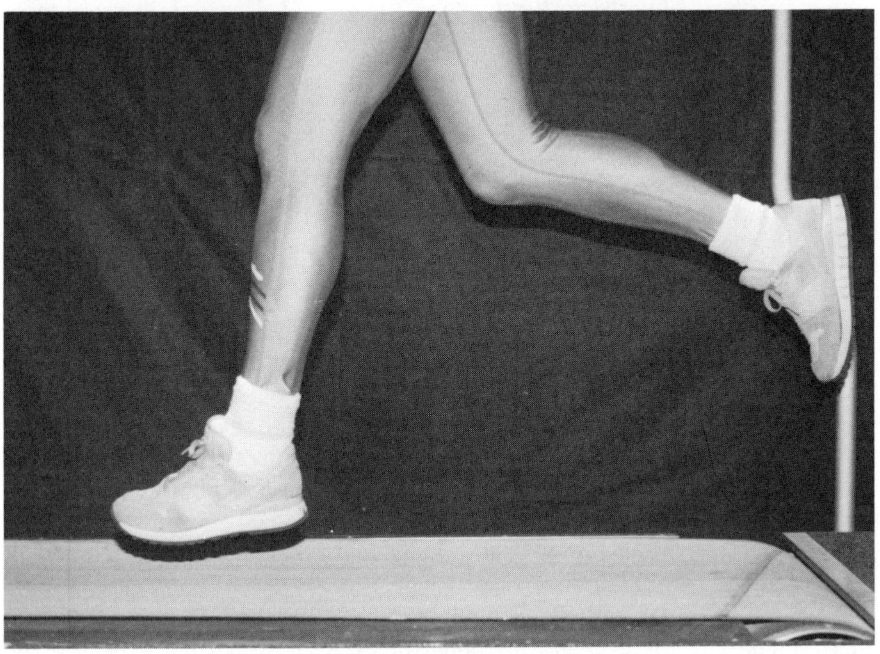

FIGURE 16. The same subject runs at a 9 MPH pace. Notice that both feet are in the air at the same time. In this particular subject, vertical deflection is rather large as there is approximately 3 to 5 inches between the left foot and the running surface.

body weight, depending on speed of movement. This means that the runner must be able to absorb some of the shock imparted to the feet. Although the ground reaction force may be three to four times body weight, the internal forces on the joint contact points and in the individual muscles may amount to about ten times body weight. There is no doubt that the "pounding" that occurs during a long-distance run such as a marathon may very well result in some form of musculoskeletal problem. Running stride, speed, body weight, foot contact area, and type of footwear all play a role in either alleviating or facilitating the effects of ground reaction force. Several studies have shown that shoes definitely play a role in reducing ground reaction forces. Unfortunately, the comparison of this variable between similar subjects and different shoes is not very elucidating.

Running Style and Form

Certainly everyone knows how to walk and run, since humans have all done these activities since childhood. However, many individuals do not know how to run properly. If you observe some good long-distance runners closely, they appear to "float" almost effortlessly along the ground. If you similarly observe some untrained or novice runners, it is evident that there is a great deal of wasted motion.

The following section summarizes optimal running conditions. Together with the photographs and figures presented, it should give a good representation of how to run most effectively and economically.

Foot Contact

This discussion analyzes the interaction between the feet and the ground during the striking phase in running. As a general rule, it can be said that in walking the heel strikes the ground first, then the remainder of the foot, and lastly the toes. As you begin running, the length of foot contact with the ground diminishes. However, many runners and even elite distance runners still hit the ground first with the heel, usually the lateral outside portion (see Figures 17, 18, and 19).

However, there is a great deal of individual variability as to which part of the foot hits the ground first, irrespective of speed. In almost every case, ground contact is made first with the lateral border of the shoe. Studies show that most runners hit the ground first along the entire posterior 60 percent of the shoe length (Cavanagh & LaFortune, 1980). Figure 20 illustrates the classification of rearfoot or midfoot strikers and the areas of the shoe bottom that are involved.

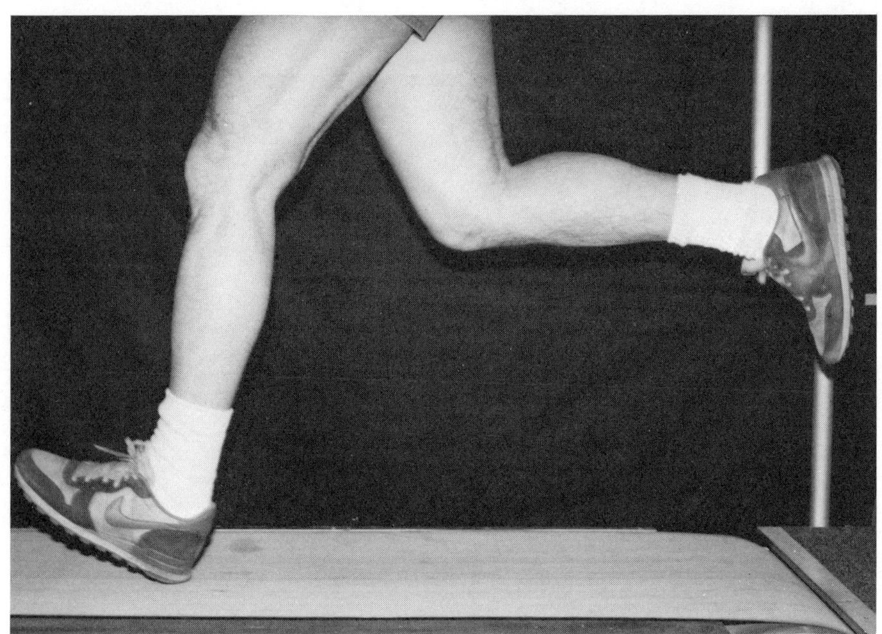

FIGURE 17. The subject displays the classic heel strike while running at a moderate pace on the treadmill. Notice that the outside border of the heel is in contact with the ground first.

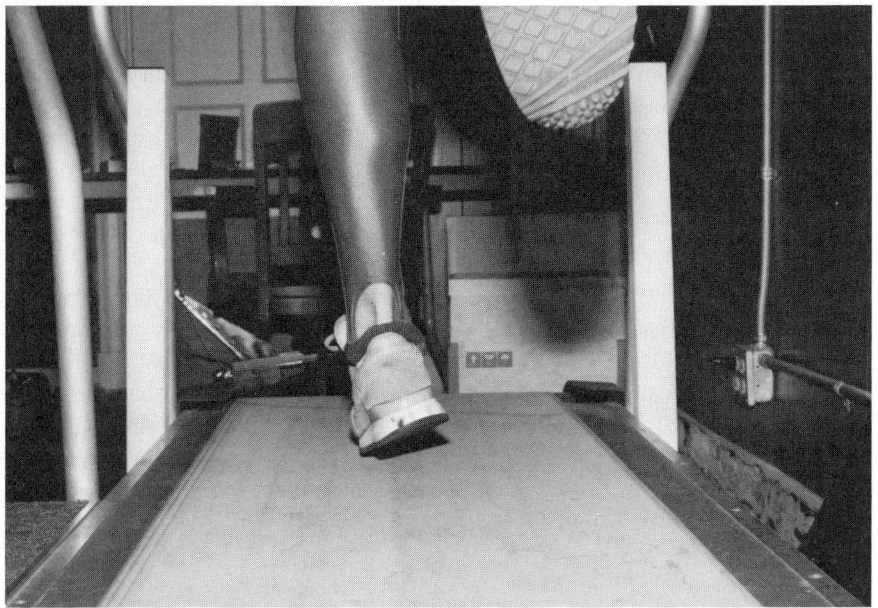

FIGURE 18. Aside from the heel strike, the lateral aspect of the foot is usually in contact with the ground first, as demonstrated by this runner.

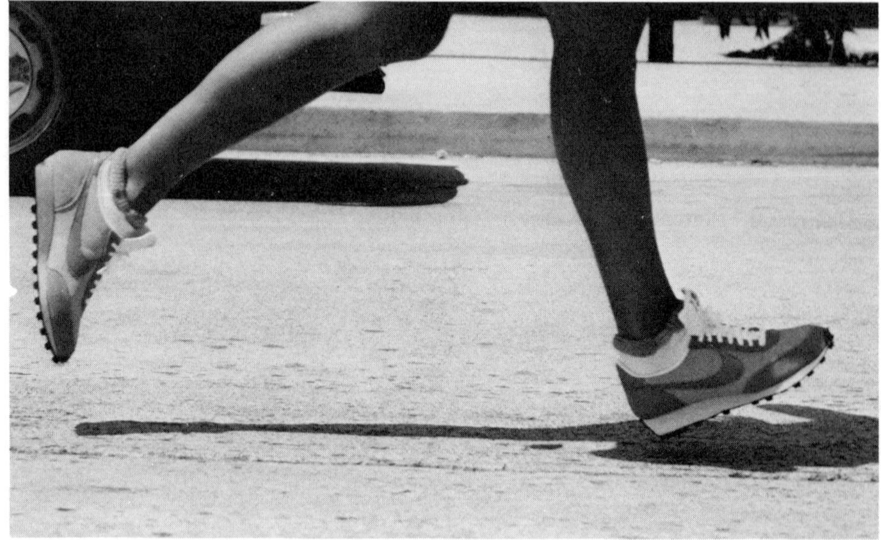

FIGURE 19. This subject, who is running outdoors, displays the classic heel strike.

Heel to Toe

Despite this degree of variability, one thing is certain: at distance-running speeds you should never land on the forepart (ball) of your foot, as you do in sprinting. Running on your toes for a long period of time can cause some severe musculoskeletal discomfort in the lower leg and knee since there is a much smaller area (and contact time) for shock absorption to take place. Most of the force is transmitted directly to the lower leg and knee. Proper running form consists of hitting lightly on the heel (or slightly in front of it) then rolling over the foot (see Figures 21 and 22).

Since the average person does not have access to high-speed motion picture analysis, how can you determine which part of your foot hits the ground first? Although it is not a very accurate method, you can determine this point by looking at the greatest wear points on the bottom of your shoes. So many runners appear to strike on the lateral aspect of the heel that some shoe manufacturers are using more durable materials in this part of the shoe. Figure 23 illustrates normal wear on the outside portion of a pair of running shoes.

Shoe Wear

Wear is caused by the relative motion between the outsole and the ground. You would not necessarily expect any relationship between the regions of maximum wear and the regions where maximum forces occur. Wear occurs during

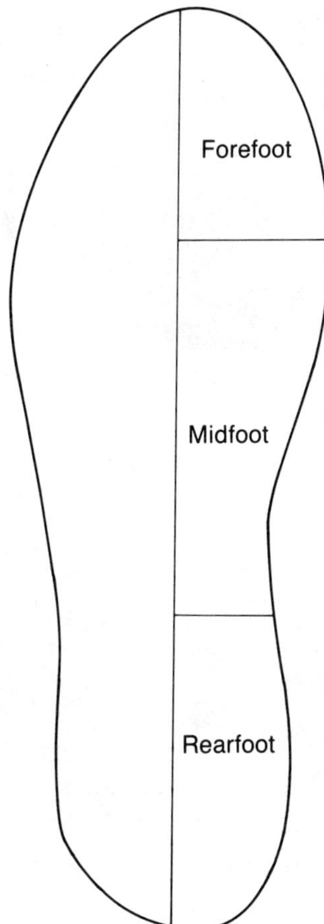

FIGURE 20. A pattern of the bottom of a foot. A recent biomechanics study indicates that the strike index (greatest force generated between foot and ground) varies considerably between runners. It appears that the greatest number of runners have a strike index from rearfoot to midfoot.

the initial scuffing at touchdown and this region usually extends over the entire posterior two-thirds of the shoe. Another major wear region is likely to be under the forefoot where the center of pressure is located during the late support phase (a slight twist occurs at this time).

From studies done on runners, it appears that the midregion and forefoot areas are where maximum vertical forces occur (Cavanagh & LaFortune, 1980). In spite of the wear and high-impact forces in these regions, most shoe manufacturers appear to have neglected building up these areas. Most of the attention has centered on building up and cushioning the heel area of shoes. There is no doubt that this area needs to be improved. However, there is also the need for

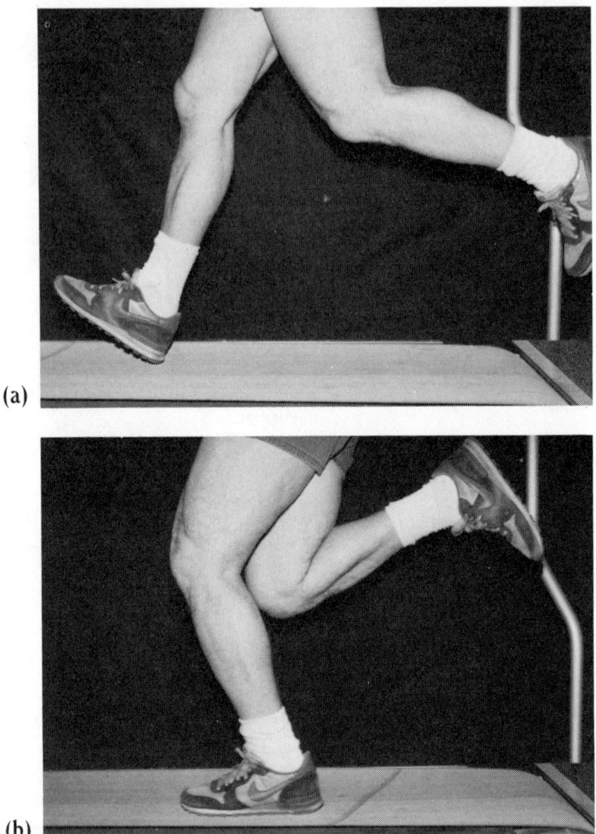

FIGURE 21. These photographs illustrate what happens from heel strike: (a) the heel hits the ground first when the entire foot comes down (b) in preparation for the push-off phase of the stride.

protection of the foot from impact in the area from the heel to 60 percent of the shoe length. Shoes should be available which will help cushion individuals in the midfoot and forefoot region, especially if an individual happens to be a midfoot striker. Unfortunately, without some form of sophisticated analysis, it would not be possible to determine initial foot contact area for an individual with reasonable accuracy.

Stride Length and Frequency

As in the previous section on foot contact, the length of the stride and the number of steps taken are quite variable. Obviously, the length of the stride is determined primarily by the length of the legs. Therefore, a tall long-legged

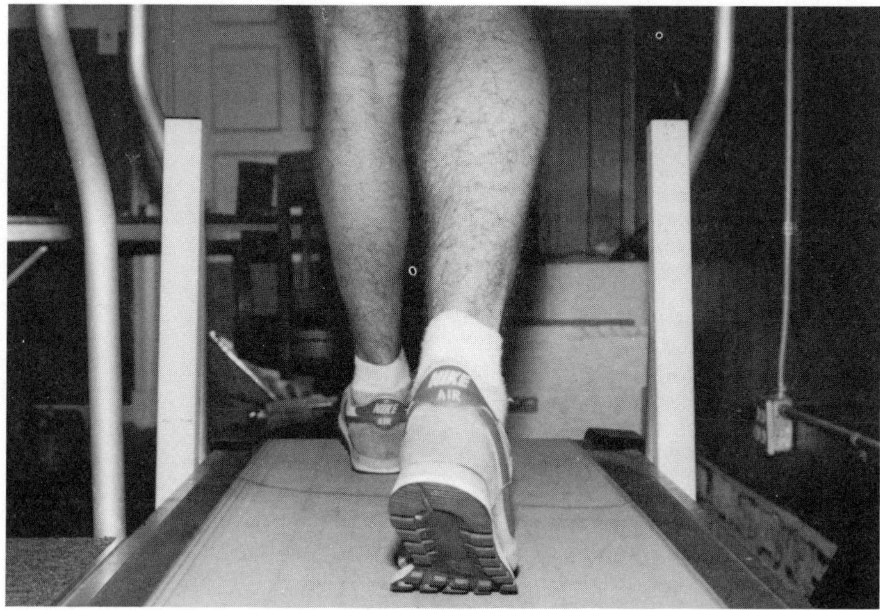

FIGURE 22. Although this subject is walking, the push-off phase of the right foot can be observed. Obviously, this is much more pronounced in running.

individual has a longer stride than a shorter person. However, within individuals of the same leg length there is often a great deal of variation in stride length. Many people inadvertently feel that a long stride is more efficient and is better running form. In fact, studies on elite distance runners show that they take medium stride lengths, but their stride frequencies are much greater (Burke, 1976; Hogberg, 1952; Pollock, 1977). Figure 24 shows the relationship between stride length and the amount of energy utilized (economy). It is clear that there is an optimal stride length for each individual which must be determined by trial-and-error approach.

Overstride

Overstriding may also result in musculoskeletal problems when individuals do it continuously, especially during long road races. The reason for this is that a longer stride results in greater hip rotation and stretching of the musculature in the groin and hip area. In addition, the increased stride results in greater vertical displacement which could lead to a greater ground reaction force on landing.

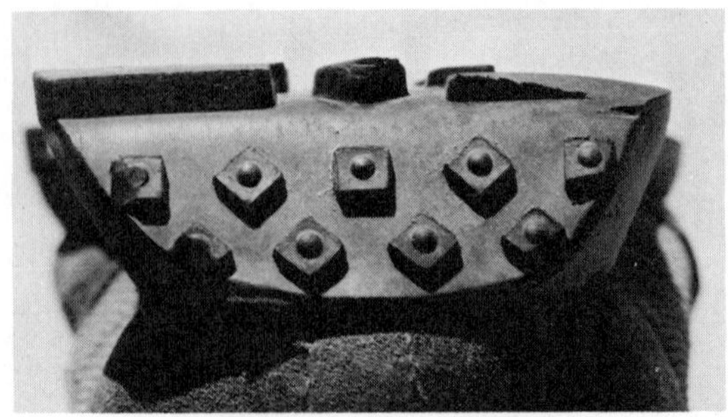

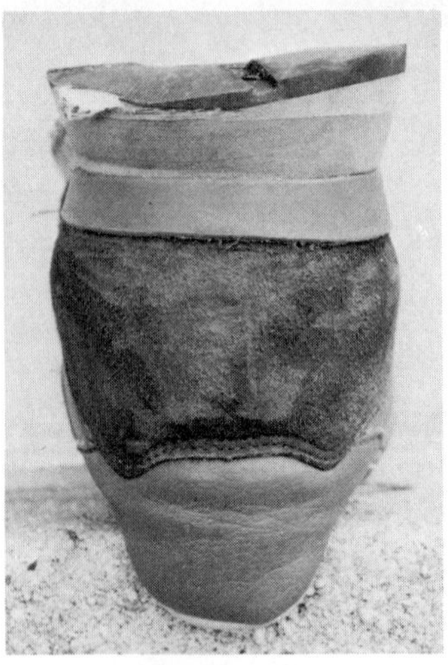

FIGURE 23. These photographs depict the bottom heel portion of two running shoes. Although they were not worn for that many miles, you can see excessive wear on the lateral border of the heel. Since the heel hits the ground first, the greatest wear is expected at this site.

Foot Alignment

One of the more common faults individuals have while running (and also when walking) is improper foot alignment. Many people walk and run with their toes pointed away, at a 45-degree angle from the midpoint of the body (see Figure 25). This is sometimes referred to as *duck walk*.

The opposite of the duck-walk style is a pigeon-toed one. This occurs when the toes point at an inward angle (not quite 45 degrees) from the midpoint (see Figure 26).

When the feet are out of alignment, the force, which is generated by the toes against the ground, is displaced side-to-side rather than straight back (see

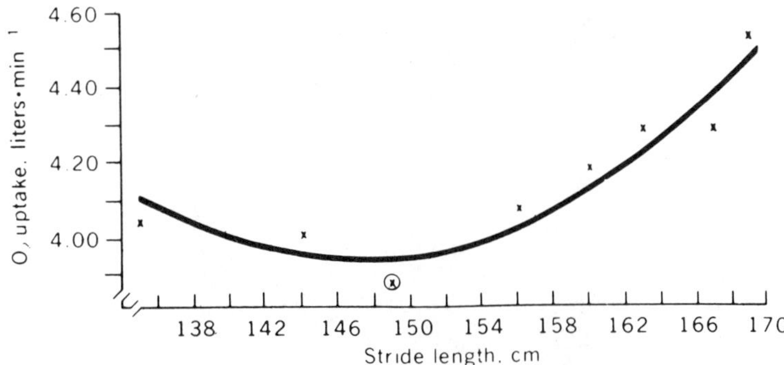

FIGURE 24. Relationship between oxygen consumption (energy expenditure) and stride length during running. ⊗ represents the chosen stride length for this runner. (From P. Hogberg, "How Do Stride Length and Stride Frequency Influence the Energy Output During Running?" *Arbeitsphysiologie* 14(1952): 437. Copyright © 1952 by Springer Verlag. Reprinted with permission.)

Figure 27). Running in this manner may also place undue strain on the knees.

One of the best methods of checking out your alignment is to run on a road or path with a center stripe about 2 to 4 inches wide. Run down the center of the stripe. The medial aspect (insides) of your feet should touch the stripe on each side. This can also be done while walking.

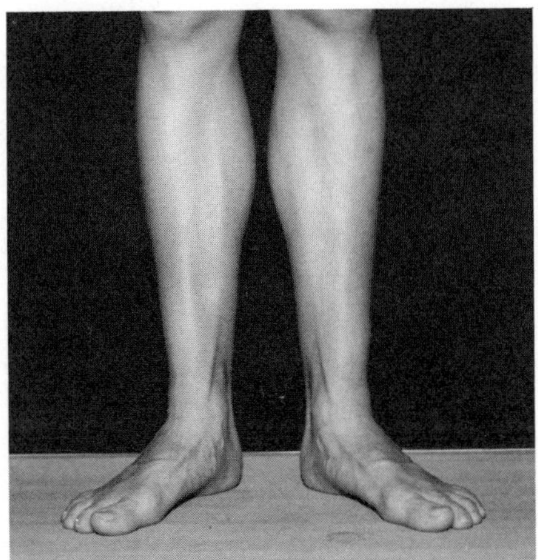

FIGURE 25. The subject is standing with feet pointed at a 45-degree angle from the midline of the body. This is commonly called a duck-walk style and many people run this way.

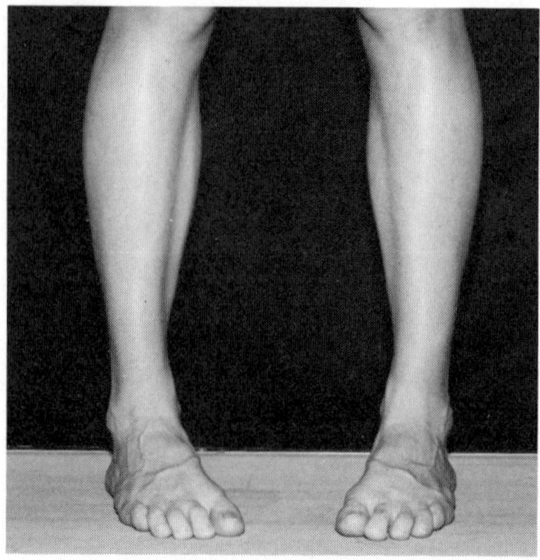

FIGURE 26. The subject demonstrates a pigeon-toed stance. Again, some individuals run with their feet pointing in this direction.

Foot and Leg Alignment

As a result of an improvement in cinematographical analysis, it has been discovered that many runners (as many as 60 percent in one study) display a rather serious foot alignment problem called *pronation* (Cavanagh, 1980). This deviation can best be visualized by observing the relationship between the foot, ankle, and lower leg in Figure 28. This is considered normal foot and leg alignment.

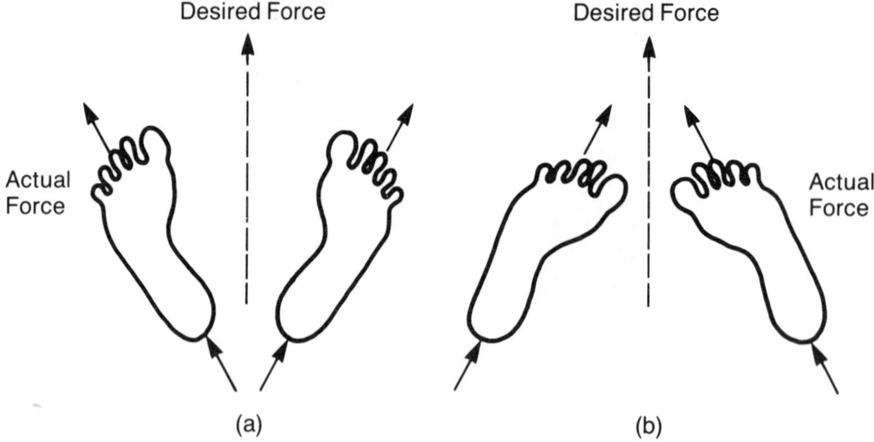

FIGURE 27. A schematic diagram of the direction of force generated during forward motion: (a) duck-walk style; (b) pigeon-toed style.

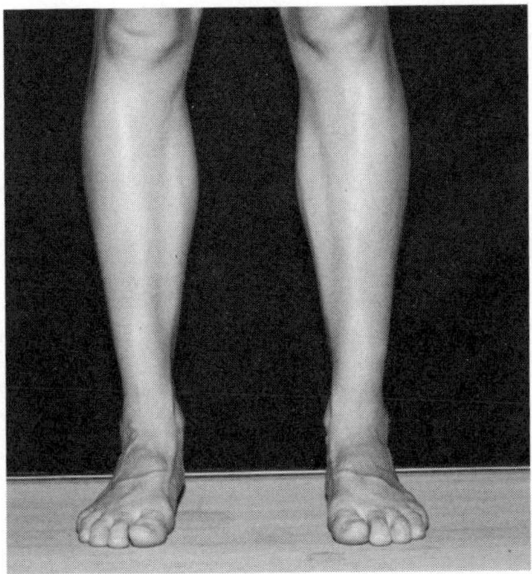

FIGURE 28. The subject stands upright displaying what is considered to be normal alignment of the feet and lower legs.

Figures 29 and 30 show a subject supinating her feet (which is somewhat common in running) and also pronating them. Excessive foot pronation may be caused by a number of factors, some of which are genetic, such as structural abnormalities in the foot. Shoes with little or no arch support may promote this condition, as well as excessively worn-out shoes. Finally, pronation may be caused by the running surface itself. If you are a road runner and the typical

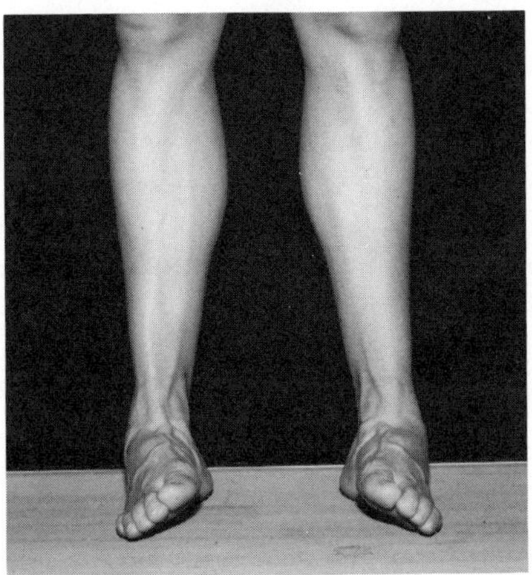

FIGURE 29. The subject demonstrates an exaggerated example of supination. The weight is on the outer (lateral) borders of the feet.

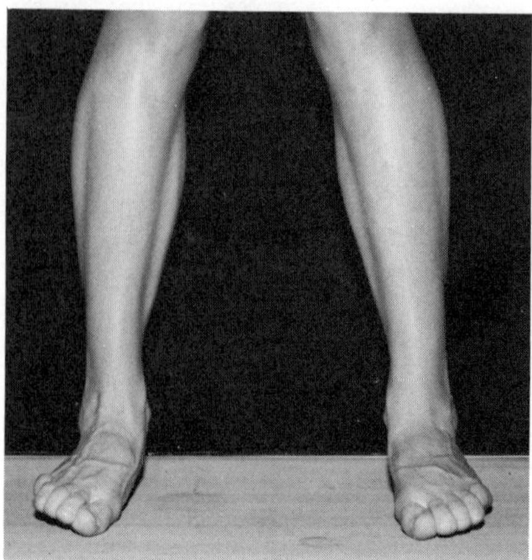

FIGURE 30. This is a classic case of pronation, which is common in runners. Although pronation occurs to varying degrees, it can lead to some rather severe orthopedic problems. Therapeutic methods are discussed in the text.

trail is by the side of the road, the foot closest to the center of the road will be pronated because of the crown in the road. This is also typical when running on a beach where the sand tilts downward toward the water.

Correcting Chronic Pronation

Chronic pronation may result in chondromalacia (pain in the knee) and shin-splints in the runner. Therefore, it is advisable to correct the condition if it exists. However, determination of the deviation is not a simple matter. High-speed photography of a runner from front and back is the best method, assuming the equipment is available. Another possibility would be to have someone well-informed about pronation and supination to run behind you and observe your feet and ankles. This method would only work if you have extreme pronation, since moderate degrees would not be visible to the naked eye. Examination of the excessive wear points on your shoes may also give you some information. However, you may have to rely on a podiatrist (foot specialist) or orthopedist.

Arm Swing and Upper Body Movement

When running, the legs move forward and backwards a substantial distance. Since the legs are connected to the pelvic bone (hip) which is in turn connected to the spine, there must be some movement in the upper trunk during running.

The function of the arms is essentially to counterbalance the movement of the hips and trunk. The arms should hang naturally at the sides, elbows bent at a 90-degree angle, palms facing inward. Arms and legs swing in opposition—that is, as the right leg moves forward the right arm moves backward (see Figure 31).

The importance of the arm swing in running can be illustrated by trying to run with your arms held at your sides. Balance under this condition is very difficult, especially at faster speeds. Arms and hands should be kept as loose as possible to prevent tension from developing in the upper shoulders and chest. During a long run, many runners display shoulder and arm fatigue, which is not unusual considering the degree of muscular involvement.

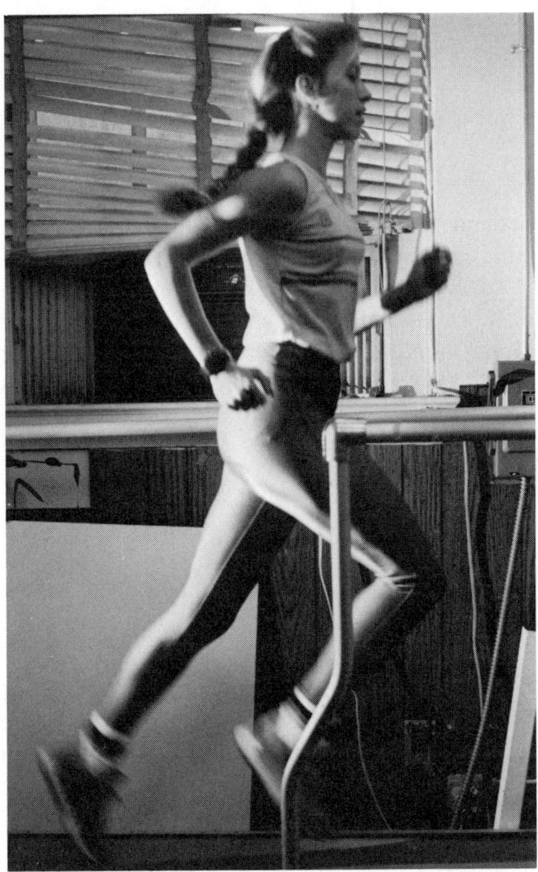

FIGURE 31. While running, the arms basically swing in opposition to the legs (on the same side) and help reduce trunk movement. Elbows are bent at a 45-degree angle, palms facing inward. This subject shows excellent arm carriage while running.

Running with Weights

A fairly common sight today is an individual running on a track or along a trail carrying small weights in each hand. These weights are usually one to five pounds and have been popularized by a text extolling the benefits to be derived from carrying weights. The implication is that running with weights simulates cross-country skiing, which is an excellent activity. There is no doubt that any extra weight a person carries while running will result in an increased caloric cost (expending more calories and therefore a greater weight loss) per mile. However, carrying weights in each hand may alter normal gait patterns and possibly result in a musculoskeletal problem. It is suggested that weight training be carried out while you are stationary and, if you wish to increase the caloric cost of your run, the simple solution would be to increase the mileage.

Summary

In reading this chapter, you must keep in mind that the concepts presented are based on sound biomechanical and physiological principles. However, this does not imply that everyone should run with exactly the same form. Studies done on elite distance runners have shown substantial variation in running form and many were found to display incorrect alignments. If the principles of good form are kept in mind during training, running will be more efficient and many of the common musculoskeletal injuries associated with long-term running programs can be avoided.

Review

1. Running results in a great deal of force being fed up through the legs from impact with the ground. The forces generated can lead to injuries (over time) if the runner does not have proper foot, leg, and trunk alignment.
2. In distance running, foot contact is made first with the lateral border of the foot in 80 percent of cases studied.
3. Stride length should be determined by the leg length and biomechanical peculiarities of the individual. Overstriding usually leads to more problems than understriding.

4. Foot pronation is one of the more serious problems a runner must cope with; before it can be modified, it must be diagnosed properly.
5. Maximizing favorable biomechanical principles to develop good running form should be implemented by anyone who has the desire to be a long-distance runner.

CHAPTER 6

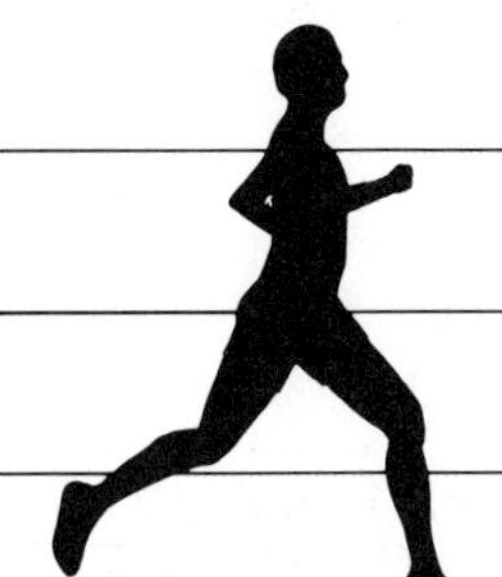

Injuries and Other Problems Associated with Running

Orthopedic Problems

If you decide to become involved in a long-distance running program, chances are very good that you will eventually develop some form of musculoskeletal difficulty. These problems may manifest themselves simply as minor pain or possibly as a severe debilitating injury. Injuries related to a running program are most often a result of what is termed *overuse syndromes*. *Overuse* refers to the chronic stress placed on the feet, legs, hips, and back, which is caused by the constant interaction of feet and ground during long-distance running. Injuries related to overuse include stress fractures, chondromalacia (pain in the knee), shinsplints, and tendonitis. Studies done on men and women participating in a jogging program indicate that the incidence of injuries is as high as 54 percent. In the 1983 New York City marathon, 500 of the 1,100 injured runners who required medical attention had complaints related to pain in the lower extremities, such as blisters, strains, and sprains (Vaughan, 1984).

Chronic Pain

As a runner, you must be able to cope with discomfort and pain, especially in very long-distance training. However, some individuals carry the "Spartan" attitude a bit too far. They continue to run despite chronic pain, and the usual outcome is that a moderate injury develops into an incapacitating one. Certainly there are some types of injuries that are not aggravated by continued running. In fact, rehabilitation may even be accelerated in certain instances by light to moderate running. The reason for this is that exercise increases blood flow to the exercising tissues. This increased circulation helps promote recovery, especially in soft-tissue injuries. You must remember that pain may be an ally because it gives you information that something is wrong. It may also be a harbinger of more serious consequences if the problem is not rectified.

An individual who continues to run, despite the injury, often adopts an abnormal running gait. For example, an individual experiencing pain in the left knee has a tendency to place more weight on the right leg during each stride. Studies done on patients who have undergone partial limb replacement indicate that much more stress is placed on the "good" leg. If the runner continues to do this, invariably he or she will develop problems in the uninjured limb. If you are injured and do not wish to experience the effects of detraining, there are alternatives to running. In general, swimming and bicycling can be performed, even though running is contraindicated. The rationale for this is that in these activities there is no "pounding" nor is there any weight-bearing by the limbs. Swimming is an almost ideal therapeutic exercise since the body is almost weightless in the water and very little stress is placed on any of the joints. If a pool is available where the water is very shallow (2 to 4 feet), you can actually run across the length of the pool while submerged in water up to your waist or neck.

Stress Fractures

The stress or fatigue fracture is not due to an acute injury (such as an impact injury), but to excessive stress (hence the name) placed on bones during typical activities, such as walking and running. Stress fractures occur during remodeling of normal bone when resorption of bone exceeds repair. Unusual physical activity causes remodeling. During remodeling, normal bone is temporarily weakened by the rapid osteoclastic resorption. When the reactive bone is inadequate for reinforcement, a break will be seen in the cortex. With further overexercise, the stress fracture can develop into a complete fracture. The bones of the foot, leg (tibia, fibula, femur), pelvis, and back are the most frequently affected, since these weight-bearing bones are subject to the most stress. This type of injury is characterized by localized, severe pain, which is accentuated by stress, such as bearing weight. It can sometimes be incorrectly diagnosed as shinsplints when it occurs in the lower leg bones (tibia or fibula). It can only be diagnosed by the meticulous examination of the X-rays taken of the affected area. Figure 32 shows a stress fracture of the tibia. The stress fracture is characterized by the lump or callus on the right side of the bone. The small fracture line can be identified as the horizontal line. This spot or callus is generally weaker than the rest of the bone and is susceptible to complete fracture if treatment is not provided. The best treatment for all stress fractures is rest from any activity that causes pain. Under some circumstances, a cast may have to be applied to the limb.

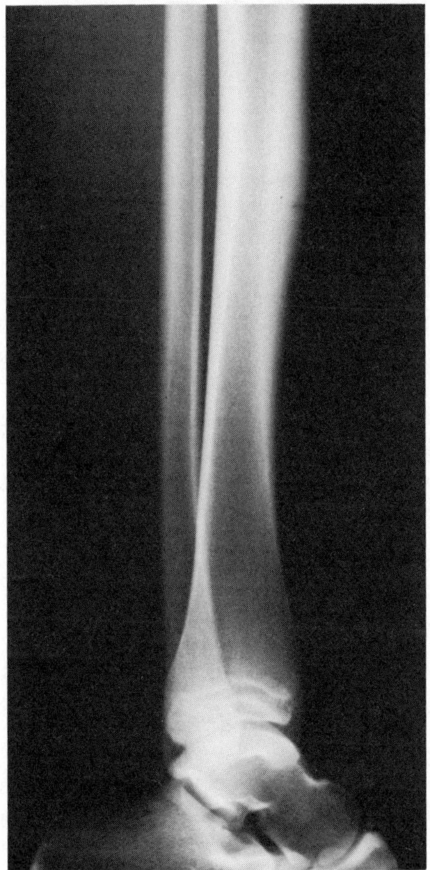

FIGURE 32. A typical stress fracture, diagnosed by X-ray examination of the lower leg. The fracture can be seen as the small horizontal line about midway up the right side of the tibia (large lower leg bone). Note the bump or callus at this spot, which is actually the proliferation of new bone in the affected area. (Photo courtesy of the Medical Photography Lab, Centinela Hospital, Inglewood, California.)

Tendonitis and Strains

Tendonitis

A tendon is the part of the muscle that attaches to a bone. Unlike the soft, fleshy muscle, the tendon is very slender and hard, almost rope-like in appearance. Tendons are subjected to wear where they pass over bony prominences. Small, fluid-filled sacs known as *bursae*, found between the tendon and the bone, cushion the tendon. Bursitis is an inflamation of the bursae. Tendonitis is usually the result of overuse, poor shoe design, and structural deviations.

Strain

This term is generally applied when there is injury to the musculotendinous unit from overuse or overstress. There are various degrees of severity related to strains. In the mildest case, there is usually local pain and tenderness which is aggravated by running. However, a severe strain indicates a rupture or separation of part of the musculotendinous unit. Sometimes the muscle separates from the tendon or the tendon pulls away from the bony insertion. In either case, the injury is almost completely incapacitating. The most common sites for these severe strains (or pulls as they are usually called) are the hamstrings and Achilles tendon. The severe strain does not usually occur in the long-distance runner; it is more commonly found in sprinters. However, it can occur during moderate running pace or perhaps during the exertion of running up or down hills.

Common Strain Sites

Achilles Tendon

Achilles tendonitis is one of the most common problems for the long-distance runner. Symptoms are usually pain and swelling in the back of the heel along the course of the tendon. Overuse, improper shoes, excessive foot pronation, and hill running are all causative factors. Problems occur when some of the following shoe designs are present: low heel, no arch support, and soft heel counter. Achilles tendonitis is especially prevalent in runners who have very tight calf muscles. This is why it is strongly suggested that a good flexibility program be incorporated into everyone's running schedule.

Treatment of tendonitis first involves identification and removal (if possible) of the causative factor(s). Changing to a pair of shoes with good arch support, heel wedge, and rigid heel counter are the simplest solutions, assuming that the present shoes were the culprits. Other solutions include reducing hill running, reducing total mileage, and adequate stretching prior to and after running.

Anterior Tibial Tendon

This tendon acts in opposition to the Achilles tendon. It functions as a *dorsiflexor of the foot* (lifting the toes up). Downhill running and excessive foot pronation can cause inflammation in this area.

Leg Adductor Muscle Group (Groin Area)

These muscles adduct (move inwards toward the groin) the upper leg and keep it in alignment. This muscle group is often overstretched in downhill running and while overstriding. Pain occurs on the inner side of the upper thigh and on the lower abdomen.

Treatment

The general first-aid treatment for a soft-tissue injury, such as a strain, includes ice and analgesics (such as aspirin). Many individuals mistakently use external heat (hot water or heating pad) for acute injuries. However, cold is the prescribed treatment, generally in the form of ice. It is a good idea to ice down a painful area after a long run. Cold tends to decrease the pain and helps prevent possible edema (fluid accumulation which can hamper recovery). As a mild analgesic (pain killer), aspirin is the most recommended drug. A suggested dosage would be two aspirin, four times per day, taken with plenty of fluid (water or juice).

Prevention

The junction strength between a tendon and bone is decreased with inactivity and increased with chronic activity (training). However, the objective of running as a training modality is to build up that strength, *gradually*. In many individuals, the sudden increase in training loads is much too rapid. As a result, a chronic strain develops. Therefore, one of the keys to prevention is to become well-conditioned, but gradually in an intelligent progression.

Shinsplints

This is a sort of "catch-all" term used to describe almost any pain in the lower leg area. Since the term does apply to different pain sites, it is difficult to identify one specific orthopedic factor. However, it appears that shinsplints are most commonly caused by an irritation of the membrane surrounding the tibial bone or at the attachments of the anterior and posterior tibial muscles.

The irritation may be a result of several factors. Some of these factors include a sudden increase in training intensity, shoes with poor cushioning, and running on hard surfaces, especially concrete. Obviously, to prevent this condition change footwear and run on a much softer surface, such as grass or composition track surfaces. Another remedy is to strengthen the lower leg muscles so that they will be better able to withstand fatigue during prolonged activity. Still another solution is to increase flexibility of the front and back muscles of the lower leg by stretching before and after running. Ice and anti-inflammatory medication are the usual treatments for shinsplint pain.

Chondromalacia

Pain in the area of the knee joint is the most common experienced by the long-distance runner. Figure 33 displays lateral and posterior X-rays of the knee joint. Illustrated are the femur, patella or kneecap, tibia, and fibula. The knee is basically a hinge joint and during running it flexes and extends. However, some rotation also occurs at the knee joint in running (which is greatly pronounced if foot pronation occurs) and this results in severe irritation along the patella. The stronger the muscles are that cross the knee (quadriceps and hamstrings), the less the rotation in this area during running.

A glance at Figure 33(a) shows that the large thigh bone (femur) rides on top of the tibia in a rocking chair style. Two pieces of cartilage (menisci) separate these two bones and help act as shock absorbers. Excessive running may very likely accelerate the normal wear that occurs in these cartilages. As a general rule, you should try to reduce the ground forces the knees must absorb. During the marathon, an average runner takes approximately 25,000 steps. As stated earlier, as the foot hits the ground during each step, ground forces of up to four times body weight will be transmitted to the limbs, and possibly the articular cartilage.

Susceptibility to Injury

A relatively strong statement was made at the beginning of this chapter regarding the incidence of injuries related to a long-distance training program. In spite of this, many individuals have been running for years and have never incurred any injuries. What factor or factors could be at work that would cause one individual to be more susceptible to injury than another? Some of these factors may be attributed to the biomechanics of running and proper shoe selection. There are probably other factors, however, over which an individual has very little control. This would concern structural abnormalities in the skeletal system.

Very few individuals are born "perfect" from the standpoint of the skeletal system. In addition, abnormal stresses placed on the skeletal system during the growth stages may permanently alter a bone in terms of shape or length. For

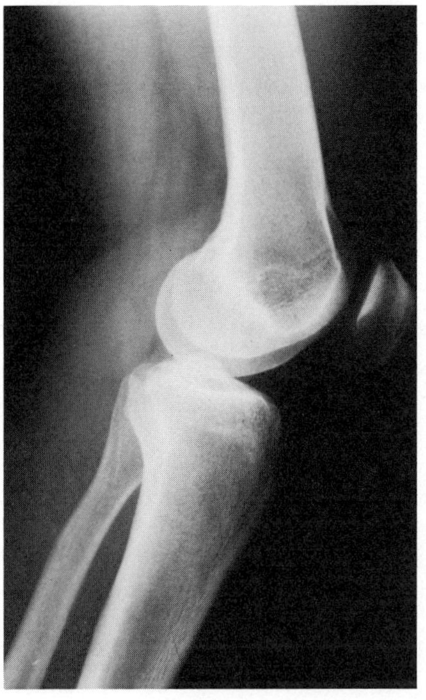

(a)

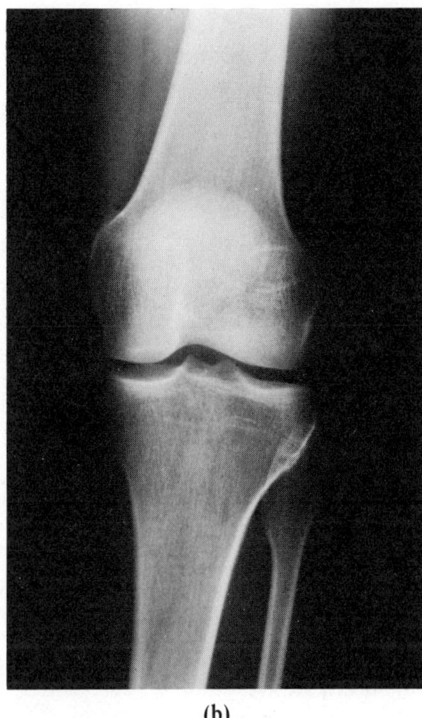

(b)

FIGURE 33. X-ray photographs of the knee joint, looking at the lateral view (a) and a posterior view (b). Visible are part of the femur (large thigh bone), patella or knee cap, tibia, and fibula. The knee joint is highly susceptible to rotational stresses during running. The inside of the patella is particularly prone to injury and degeneration in long-distance runners. (Photos courtesy of the Medical Photography Lab, Centinela Hospital, Inglewood, California.)

example, gymnasts typically develop certain spinal deviations (i.e., lordosis) that are often permanent. An individual may have broken a leg bone and had it casted for several months, with the possible end result of developing a shorter bone length in one leg. These are just a few of the many possible situations that could develop.

In many runners, one leg may be slightly shorter than the other. This difference is imperceptible to the untrained eye, but the end result is a lateral spinal deviation (scoliosis). Since the leg is connected to the pelvic bone and this in turn is connected to the spinal column, leg problems often cause injuries to the back. Some individuals have (genetically) an abnormally short big toe. This almost guarantees that the person will pronate his or her foot during running, unless some type of shoe orthotics are available. Again, these are just a few of the possible implications resulting from skeletal differences. In running, the feet hit the ground many times over a long period of time. Therefore, small problems that normally would not surface during normal walking are highly evident during a long run. For example, if one ran for one hour at a 6-minutes per mile pace, each foot would hit the ground approximately 5,000 times! If there was even the slightest structural or functional deviation, problems would invariably develop.

Miscellaneous Problems

Blisters

Everyone who has run has developed blisters on the feet. Blisters are usually created from excessive abrasion or trauma to the skin. This can be caused by poorly fitting shoes, poorly fitting socks (or socks that tend to bunch up or fold), and also from improper biomechanics (i.e., foot pronation). However, blisters almost always develop on the feet when you run for a long period of time, even with good shoes, socks, and biomechanics. You might say that blisters are an "occupational hazard" associated with running. They can be very painful and at times may force a runner to drop out of a race. Treatment includes sterile laceration (rub area with alcohol or other topical antiseptic), pressure to remove fluid, and leaving the outer layer of skin in place. Sometimes special Band-aids can be used to prevent the outer layer of skin from being torn away and to keep the area relatively clean and dry. Vaseline can sometimes be used as a preventive measure. You should rub it on areas of your feet that have been traditional sore spots in the past. You should never wear a brand new pair of running shoes on a very long run. This would almost guarantee the development of painful blisters. You should break in the new shoes gradually, with shorter runs before trying them on a very long run or a race.

Toe Problems

The toes are very often traumatized during long-distance running. Each time the foot hits the ground, the toes are jammed forward. If the toe box in the shoes is not wide enough (there is a great deal of variability in width of both shoes and feet) or if there is insufficient room in front, the toes are jammed against the shoe. Over a long period of time, blisters, callouses, and hammertoes (bent over toes) will develop. It is suggested that, in addition to properly fitting shoes, you trim your toenails before a long run. When long toenails are jammed, it usually results in the death and loss of the nail.

Athlete's Foot

Another common medical problem for athletes is the condition known as athlete's foot or, more accurately, *tinea pedia*. This is actually a fungal infection of the foot. Fungal infections can occur anywhere on the body. Fungi grow best in unsanitary conditions, combined with warmth, moisture, and darkness. The organism is commonly called *ringworm* or *tinea* and is classified according to the area of the body infected. Spores of these fungi are extremely contagious and may be spread by direct contact, contaminated clothing, or dirty locker rooms and showers. Susceptibility to fungal infections such as athlete's foot depends on several factors:

Individual's immune response mechanism. Some individuals are highly resistant to certain fungal infections, whereas others are not. This is similar to other infectious diseases.

Coming into contact with the infectious organisms. Some individuals may never become exposed to these fungi.

Using good preventive measures. Keeping your feet dry and using talcum powder after showering is a good practice. Always wearing clean white socks and avoiding dirty shower room facilities also helps.

Treatment for athlete's foot includes the use of fungicidal powders or creams. Feet and toes must be kept dry and clean at all times. However, if the infection continues you should see a qualified dermatologist (doctor who specializes in diseases of the skin) so that successful treatment can be implemented.

Special Concerns for Young Runners

Young children and growing teenagers are not necessarily more injury prone than adults but there are some unusual circumstances that should be kept in mind when evaluating possible injuries in this population. Bones are formed from softer cartilaginous tissue, which becomes completely ossified as one gets older (about 21 years of age). A muscle attaches to a bone (insertion) at a cartilaginous point. If a great deal of stress is placed on that muscle, tendon, and bone before the cartilage ossifies, a severe inflammatory reaction could result. In extreme situations, the muscle can actually tear from the bone at this weakened point. A young runner should be aware of the possibility of such an injury, which must be diagnosed by X-ray examination. In general, young immature bones may be more susceptible to overuse injury although there is little data to support the fact that children should not run.

Testosterone and estrogen, the male and female sex hormones, are important factors in the ossification of bone. Therefore, sexually immature (from a sex hormone point of view) males and females may be more susceptible to the injuries just mentioned. Female athletes may be extremely vulnerable since it is not uncommon for very lean women to lose menstrual function temporarily (with an accompanying decrease in circulating estrogen).

Obtaining Care

Injuries are often the unwelcome consequence of a long-distance running program. Some of the more common types of injuries, their cause, prevention, and treatment were mentioned. However, this chapter is certainly not a complete discussion of the problems you may encounter as a result of running. It is suggested that you seek out some of the excellent texts available on the market dealing with sports injuries. An excellent example is by Don O'Donaghue, *Treatment of Injuries to Athletes* (1976).

The following physicians and other medical personnel are available should you need medical care:

Orthopedist. A medical doctor who specializes in the treatment of musculoskeletal disorders.

Podiatrist (D.P.M.). The podiatrist diagnoses and treats diseases and deformities of the feet or tries to prevent their occurrence. Education includes four years at a college of podiatry, after at least two years of college work. Podiatrists must pass a state board examination to obtain a license to practice.

Chiropractor (D.C.). The chiropractic method of healing is based on the theory that most human ailments or diseases are the results of the displacement of the vertebrae of the spinal column, resulting in abnormal pressure on the nerves. The chiropractic method of treatment is purely manual and never resorts to drugs or surgery. Recent practices include prescribing nutritional supplementation, heat, light, exercise, etc. Education includes at least two years of college study, four years at a chiropractic college, and passing a state licensing exam.

Athletic trainer. This individual has had training in the treatment and prevention of all types of athletic injury. The trainer usually works closely with a physician (often an orthopedist) and is associated with an athletic team or program (i.e., school or university, professional athletic team, etc.).

Physical therapist. The physical therapist (P.T.) usually has had at least one or two years of special training beyond the standard four-year college degree. The training is often specifically aimed at patients and handicapped individuals. However, the P.T. has an excellent background in dealing with musculoskeletal injuries. Many athletic trainers have a degree in physical therapy.

Dealing with Injury

Athletic injuries are often very frustrating to the individuals who have them. They may prevent the individual from running, or at least cause severe pain during the exercise. The frustration usually comes from the inability of trained personnel to successfully treat the injury. Sometimes the injury cannot even be diagnosed correctly. This is not an attempt to make excuses for the medical profession but the diagnosis and treatment of musculoskeletal injuries are extremely difficult. One of the reasons is that soft-tissue injuries (ligaments, tendons, and muscles) do not show up on X-ray examinations, for the most part. Another reason is the patients themselves. Most runners (athletes in general) expect the physician to give them something (drug, antibiotic, etc.) that will clear up the problem and allow them to maintain their training. Most individuals do not want to accept the fact that, in order for the injury to heal (in many cases), they must stop running. The final aspect is that sports injuries in general are a relatively new area for the medical community. Many physicians have never dealt with these problems before. In the event of an injury, visit a physician or medical group that deals specifically with sports medicine. These individuals would have the greatest expertise in this area.

Summary

The majority of individuals who run, at one time or another, will experience some form of injury. These injuries are most commonly categorized as overuse syndromes due to chronic stress. For the most part, rest, or a different form of exercise, is the only treatment for these types of injuries. Contributing factors for overuse injuries include high mileage training, hard road surfaces, footwear, gait anomalies, and muscle strength, among others. Acute injuries, such as muscle strains and sprains, are not common in distance runners but when they do occur should be treated with rest, ice, and anti-inflammatory drugs. Qualified medical treatment can be obtained from physicians, athletic trainers, physical therapists, podiatrists, and chiropractors.

Review

1. Overuse injuries are common problems for distance runners. This category of injury includes stress fractures, chondromalacia, shinsplints, and tendonitis.
2. Treatment for overuse injuries includes rest, changing footwear and/or running surface, a stretching and strengthening program, and anti-inflammatory drugs.
3. Continued running, with any form of lower extremity injury, is contraindicated.
4. Acute, soft-tissue injuries, such as strains and sprains, are uncommon in distance runners but should be treated with ice and analgesics.
5. Blisters of the feet are quite common in runners. Proper footwear, socks, and lubricants may help reduce the incidence of this problem.
6. Problems may occur in children and teenagers who run a great deal, and may be associated with testosterone and estrogen secretion.
7. Physicians, trainers, therapists, podiatrists, and chiropractors are all qualified to deal with running-related injuries.

CHAPTER 7

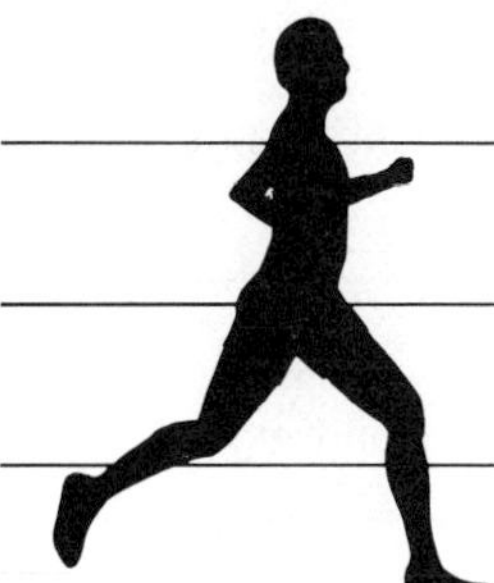

Nutritional Guidelines for the Runner

Concepts of Caloric Balance

As was stated in the introduction, one of the major afflictions of the American population, and a reason why many take up running, is the problem of being overweight. An understanding of caloric balance is crucial if you are to make any gains in weight reduction (or weight gain). All the foods you eat, and most drinks, have potential food energy or calories (Cal). An apple has about 80 Cal, a plain doughnut 160 Cal, and a Big Mac hamburger 540 Cal. The total food and drink you consume in one day determines your caloric intake. During the same time period, the body expends energy or calories. Energy is used for such processes as breathing, digestion, nerve conduction, and, of course, exercise. This total represents the caloric expenditure. The interrelationship between intake and expenditure determines changes in body weight as described in Figure 34.

The three basic fuels that supply calories are fats, proteins, and carbohydrates. Table 2 shows the amount of calories supplied by each of the three food categories. It is obvious that fats are very high in calories, and the term *high caloric density* is usually applied to foods that contain a large proportion of fat (i.e., creams, oils, nuts, cheese, high fat meats). When you lose or gain weight, the tissue change is not 100 percent fat. That is, if you lose 5 pounds, it is very unlikely that the 5 pounds is entirely fat. Some of the tissue may be glycogen (stored carbohydrate) as well as protein and some water. Unfortunately, the proportion of tissue losses that occur from individual to individual cannot be determined. As a general rule, exercise appears to increase the proportion of fat loss. Therefore, if you are trying to reduce, it would be wise to diet and exercise at the same time.

1. Caloric Intake = Caloric Expenditure

   Subject is said to be in caloric balance and no tissue weight changes should occur.

2. Caloric Intake > Caloric Expenditure

   Subject is said to be in positive caloric balance and will gain weight.

3. Caloric Intake < Caloric Expenditure

   Subject is said to be in negative caloric balance, or caloric deficit, and will lose weight.

FIGURE 34. The concept of caloric balance as it relates to weight.

Diet and Exercise

In order to lose one pound of tissue, you must burn approximately 3500 calories. This number represents a weight loss combination of approximately 70 percent fat and 30 percent protein and carbohydrate. As an example, if you would like to lose 5 pounds of weight, you must create a caloric deficit of 17,500 Cal. Since the average male may expend a total of about 3000 Cal per day (a female expends about 2200 Cal per day), it would take six days of starvation for the loss to occur. This sounds rather ridiculous, and of course it is. The present calculations are included in order to make a point. When you plan to lose weight, you must do it gradually, over a long period of time, creating an average daily caloric deficit of no more than 500 Cal. This is especially important if you are running daily (or doing other activities). Most nutritionists support this recommendation. Caloric deficits of more than 500 Cal per day could put an undue strain on the body.

TABLE 2

Fuel	*Calories/gram*	*Calories/pound*
Protein	4.0	1800
Carbohydrate	4.0	1800
Fat	9.1	4100

Individual Differences

Caloric expenditure varies considerably from individual to individual. In some small, sedentary females, total (24 hours) expenditure may amount to only 1000 Cal; whereas in some large, very active males a value of 8000 to 9000 Cal per day is not unheard of. Although the size of the person influences caloric expenditure, the most important variable is work or exercise. You can afford to eat a lot of food if you do enough exercise to expend those calories. On the other hand, if you do little more than sit all day long, even minimal amounts of food will cause weight gain. People often complain that they gain weight even though they eat "like a bird." If it is true that their caloric intake is very low and they are gaining weight, the solution must be that caloric expenditure is even lower.

The average person, even someone involved in regular exercise programs, is usually misinformed in terms of the caloric equivalents of exercise. Most people tend to overestimate the caloric value of most activities. Unfortunately, these misconceptions are perpetuated by commercial advertising which has a vested interest in selling a product or diet. Table 3 gives the caloric equivalent of some popular activities. For a more thorough and interesting comparison of caloric values, you are referred to a book entitled *Energy Equivalents of Food* by Frank Konishi.

Calorie Loss in Running

In general, the caloric equivalent of running is approximately 100 Cal per mile. Variation from this value results from differences in body weight, efficiency (economy), and speed of movement. However, for the sake of simplicity, you can use the figure of 100 Cal per mile. If you were to go out now and run 4 miles, the total expenditure would amount to approximately 400 Cal. This value is almost equivalent to a healthy slice of apple pie—without the ice cream! The point to be made here is that if you exercise by running a few miles a day you must still be careful about the quality and quantity of food you ingest. Although exercise is beneficial in maintaining body weight, you must still be very careful about dietary intake.

Water Loss in Exercise

Another important concept related to exercise and weight control is what happens to total body weight after a vigorous bout of exercise, such as running. Many individuals have experienced rather large decreases in body weight after an acute (single) bout of heavy exercise. Losses of up to 2 to 3 pounds are not unusual. However, considering what has previously been stated about the caloric equivalent of tissue and exercise, these losses appear to be irreconcilable with what is

TABLE 3. Caloric Value of Some Sports and Activities.

Remember that these are relative values. The harder or more vigorously the activity is performed, the greater the caloric expenditure.

Activity	*Cal/min/kg**
Basketball	0.138
Circuit-training	0.185
Cooking	0.048
Cycling	
5.5 MPH	0.064
9.4 MPH	0.100
Eating	0.023
Football	0.132
Golf	0.085
Lying	0.022
Running	
11:30/mile	0.135
8 min/mile	0.208
6 min/mile	0.252
Skiing—uphill	0.274
Squash	0.212
Swimming, fast crawl	0.128
Tennis	0.109

* 1 kilogram = 2.2 pounds
Source: Data taken from W. D. McArdle, F. I. Katch, and V. L. Katch, *Exercise Physiology*. Philadelphia PA: Lea & Febiger, 1986.

known. What many individuals are not aware of is that the human body is composed of approximately 60 percent water (by weight). Therefore, a 150-pound individual would have about 90 pounds of water weight. Over a short period of time, this water weight is somewhat variable. Through perspiration and/or urination, it is quite common to lose 2 to 4 pounds in a short period of time.

During a long-distance run, lasting an hour or longer, it is quite common to lose 1 to 2 liters of sweat, which would amount to about 2 to 4 pounds in body weight. Sweat rate increases dramatically if the ambient (environmental) temperature is elevated, say to 80 degrees F or higher. However, it should be pointed out that this is water weight and not *tissue* loss and eventually the weight will be regained when you ingest some fluid.

Weight Control

Weight control is a relatively simple procedure for some individuals who appear to be able to maintain a constant and normal body weight throughout their lives. For many others, however, weight control is a chronic problem that results in a great deal of unhappiness and ill health. It is not the intent of this chapter to present solutions to a problem that many feel is unsolvable, at least once adulthood is reached. However, the concepts presented here should give you some knowledge about the problems of being overweight and possibly allow you to deal with small fluctuations in body weight.

Body Composition

A discussion on weight control would not be complete without a section on the components that make up the total body weight—fat and *lean body weight* (LBW). The lean body weight of an individual is comprised of the muscles and all organs and tissues of the body (i.e., bone, nerves, blood, heart, liver, etc.). The skeletal muscles make up the largest component of the LBW, about 48 percent by weight. Many active individuals (especially muscular ones) find that they are overweight by standard height/weight tables (Metropolitan Life Insurance Tables), and yet they do not appear to be fat. This is where the differences between being overweight and being obese enter into the discussion.

Height-Weight: Body Fat

If an individual is overweight then basically that person is too heavy for his or her height. However, if an individual is classified as being obese, then he or she has too much body fat. The two conditions are not always synonymous. When an individual exercises regularly, the LBW (primarily muscle) increases, and since this tissue has a greater density (mass per unit of volume) as compared to fat, then the height/weight ratio decreases. It is certainly not unhealthy or undesirable to possess a large LBW; in fact, for many athletes a high LBW would be highly desirable, independent of their weight. Unfortunately, body weight scales give no information as to body composition. There are some fairly accurate tests available but they require laboratory facilities. Many universities, colleges, and now commercial fitness testing enterprises have the facilities to measure body composition, for a small fee. The most accurate method of assessing body composition is by *hydrostatic weighing* (see Figure 35). It is well worth both the time and expense to have this parameter measured since it is very likely to change with a program of running.

Estimating Body Fat

There are some other techniques that can be used to estimate relative body fat, although they are rather crude. First, you can use the "mirror test." This technique requires you to look at yourself in a full-length mirror, with no clothes on. If your abdomen is soft and sags over, if there is a lot of excess tissue above or below the hips, and if you can grab a handful of skin and subcutaneous tissue (fat) away from your thighs, these are all signs of obesity. Another method is the buoyancy test. While in a fresh water pool, try blowing all the air from your lungs (while in the deep end of the pool). If you sink immediately, you have *negative buoyancy*. This means that body density is greater than water (1.00 grams/cc) and, therefore, body fat may not be too high. However, if you do not sink, you have *positive buoyancy*—body density is less than water and

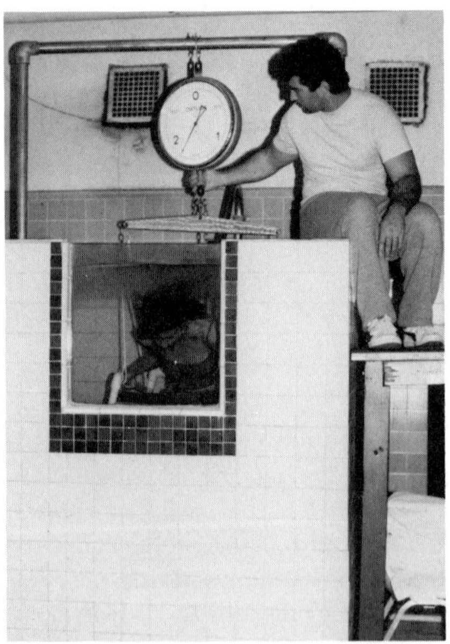

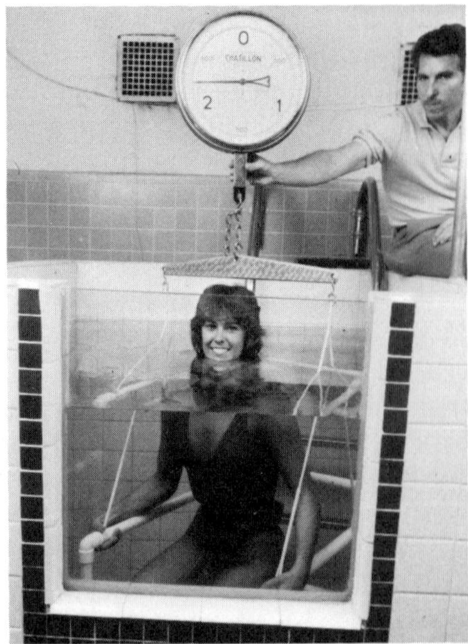

FIGURE 35. The hydrostatic weighing technique for the measurement of body composition is one of the most accurate available. The subject is weighed under water in a small tank while exhaling all of the air in the lungs.

TABLE 4. Body Fat Measurements in Normal, College-Age Males and Females.

Essential fat is considered the amount the body must have (found in bone marrow, myelin sheaths, cell membranes, etc.) to survive. Minimal fat is the lowest value that is usually found in very lean males and females. We usually expect average % fat values to increase with age.

	Average % Fat	*Normal % Fat Range*	*Essential % Fat*	*Minimal % Fat*	*Obesity % Fat*
Males (age, 17–30 yrs)	15	10–20	1–3	1–3	>20
Females (age, 17–30 yrs)	25	20–30	1–3	10–12	>30

you probably have a great deal of body fat. It should be emphasized that these techniques are merely qualitative assessments and should not replace the hydrostatic measure if available.

How much body fat does the average male or female possess? Table 4 indicates the normal ranges in body fat for college-age males and females, as well as minimal and essential fat totals. *Essential fat* is fat found in the bone marrow, cell membranes, and myelin sheaths of the nerves, among others. Minimal fat in women appears to be related to the reproductive function. The 10 percent difference in body fat between men and women is a major handicap for females in activities such as running. Studies on elite male long-distance runners indicate body fat of only 4 to 5 percent. In long-distance running, any excess weight (fat) is a disadvantage and the more successful athletes have very little of it.

Female Body Composition

As a result of becoming more competitive in long-distance running, the body compositions of these females have approached those of the male runners. Several female distance runners have been found to have body fat measurement in the 5 to 7 percent range. It would appear that, as women train harder and run longer distances, they become much leaner.

However, for many women, the advantage of being leaner (for running) may be offset by menstrual irregularities. There have been numerous cases of amenorrhea in female runners, as well as other very lean woman athletes (i.e., gymnasts, dancers). The specific cause of this problem has not been determined as yet. However, it is apparently a result of hypothalamic and/or pituitary gonadotropic hormone deficiencies. In many women who suffer from menstrual problems, there are two important factors. One is the concept of minimal fat as expressed by Dr. Albert Behnke. He stated that minimal fat in women is approximately 10 to 12 percent, the implication being that falling below this minimal value may result in menstrual dysfunction. The other factor is related to the number of total miles the woman runs. Perhaps the menstrual irregularities are a result of the large amount of energy expended while running (or doing other activities) many miles per day. Other female athletes who participate in very prolonged and heavy workouts exhibit similar results (i.e., gymnasts, swimmers, rowers, dancers). It should also be mentioned that very young female athletes (pubertal age—about 12 to 14 years) who are very lean display delayed menses or complete absence for several years.

It is unfortunate that leanness in some women is related to menstrual irregularities, because there is little doubt that low body fat is an advantage in distance running. There is no evidence, at this time, that amenorrhea is a health hazard. The short-term consequence would be lack of ovulation or infertility (and even this is not certain), which should not be a problem for the young female athlete. The long-term consequences have not been, as yet, properly evaluated.

Fundamentals of a Sound Diet

All human organisms require the following substances in varying amounts: calories (supplied by carbohydrates, fats, or proteins), proteins, vitamins, minerals, and water. They all serve vital functions and long-term deficiency of any one of them eventually leads to death. Fundamental knowledge of nutrition is based on a thorough understanding of these five factors.

Calories

The concept of caloric balance was discussed earlier. The body requires a daily supply of calories which varies depending upon age, sex, size, and physical activity. In general, carbohydrates (CHO) and fats are the primary fuel foods the cells prefer, although proteins are also catabolized for energy. In general, during a long-distance run, where you are not moving at top speed, your body will derive about half the energy from fat and the other half from CHO. The faster you run, or the closer to your maximum that you exercise, the greater the contribution from CHO.

Carbohydrates

Most runners are aware of the importance of CHO in the diet. However, you should be aware of the fact that the body has the capability of converting protein into CHO. You could survive without CHO but it would be very difficult and your physical performance would definitely be detrimentally affected. As early as the 1930s, Christensen (1931) discovered that individuals eating a high CHO diet, as compared to a fat plus protein diet (80 to 90 percent of calories from CHO) had a much greater endurance capacity on a bicycle ergometer. Since that time, many other studies have substantiated the importance of CHO in endurance performance, especially running (Bergstrom, Ahlborg, Ekelund, & Hultman, 1957; Issekutz, Birkhead, & Rodahl, 1963; Hermansen, Hultman, & Saltin, 1967).

Carbohydrate Storage

The body stores CHO in the form of glycogen, primarily in the liver and muscle cells. An average person may have a total of 500 grams available. In addition, there are approximately 5 grams of glucose available in the blood. The total value of this stored CHO is approximately 2000 calories. Compared to the almost limitless supply of calories from stored fat, the total CHO amount is relatively small. It is mainly for this reason that most experts tend to promote CHO ingestion, above all other fuels, especially prior to major races. During runs of less than 10 miles, the ingested food does not make a difference since the available glycogen is more than sufficient to meet energy demands. However, during very long runs, such as the marathon, the food you eat can be very critical.

Starch and Sugar

Carbohydrates are digested and absorbed rapidly and may get into the bloodstream in less than one hour from time of ingestion. Thus, foods that contain CHO are ideal as pre-exercise meals. Carbohydrates are classified as starches or sugars. Starches are found in foods such as grains (wheat, rye, barley, corn, rice, etc.), vegetables, beans, and fruits. Sugars, unfortunately, are found in almost everything: fruits, cakes and pastries, soft drinks, candy, chocolate, and breakfast cereals, among many others.

It is recommended that about 50 to 60 percent of your daily caloric intake come from CHO. The typical American consumes only about 45 percent of his or her calories from CHO, at this time. To make matters even worse, the typical American consumes more than half (about 52 percent) of the calories from CHO as sugars. Although sugar does supply calories, few other nutrients are contributed. The average consumption of total sugars (technically classified as sweeteners) in the United States amounts to approximately 130 pounds per person per year—a value that must be decreased.

Carbohydrate Loading

Almost anyone involved in distance running, especially marathons, has heard something about a technique called CHO loading. Basically, it is a method that has been shown to drastically increase (50 to 150 percent higher) the glycogen stores in the muscle cells. Figure 36 displays the experimental program that usually takes seven days. Many runners have utilized this method, some with good success. However, it should not be attempted by everyone, especially novice runners. Many runners do not recover sufficiently from the exhaustive run that is mandatory on the first day. For others the tremendous change in diet (90 percent fat plus protein, then 90 percent CHO) has a very detrimental effect. If you are interested in increasing your glycogen stores prior to a long race, a more rational approach woud be to complete a long run about one week prior to competition, then eat normally for the next five days. On days 6 and 7, load up on CHO. Even this toned-down program should be attempted in practice first, rather than initiating it in competition.

Fats

From the standpoint of calories, fats contribute almost half of our daily energy needs. Dietary fat makes up about 45 percent of our daily caloric intake. This value can be compared to the dietary intake of individuals living in the Orient

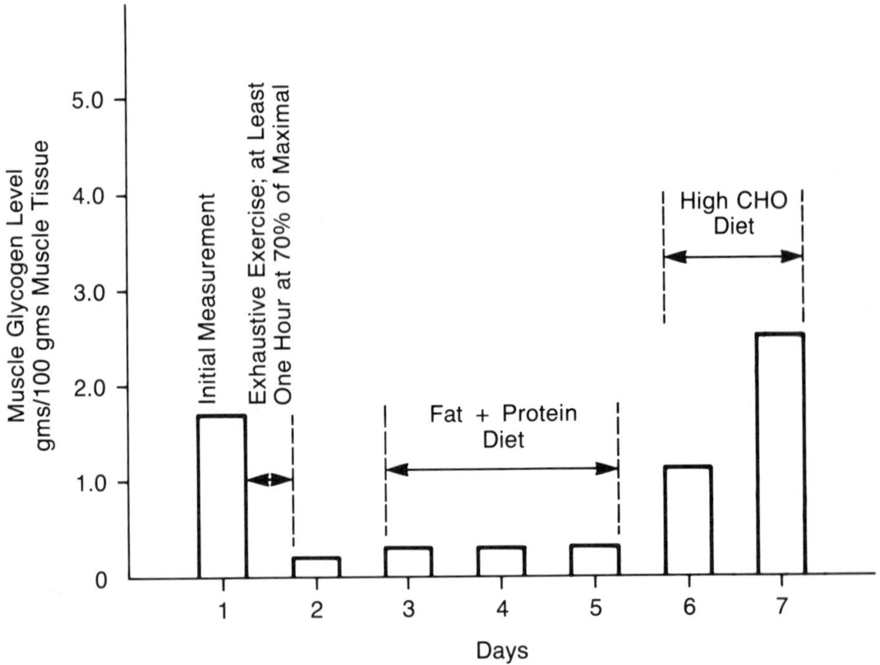

FIGURE 36. Muscle glycogen level in quadriceps (front thigh muscle) muscle of a subject before and after CHO loading experiment. An initial exhaustive exercise is mandatory to deplete glycogen stores in that specific muscle.

where only about 10 percent of ingested calories are from fat. Fat is a food of the affluent people and cultures of the world. Individuals on a lower socioeconomic scale usually cannot afford to purchase meats and dairy products, which are typically high in fat. Their diet is usually high in plant foods such as grains and vegetables.

Does the human body really need fat and is it essential for survival? There is one nutrient in fat called *linoleic acid*, which the body must have. In addition, it is the medium through which the fat-soluble vitamins are transported. However, the essential nutrients could be supplied with only 5 to 10 percent dietary fat, let alone the 45 percent that most Americans ingest. One could argue that fats are a compact and readily available source of calories. However, the problem for most Americans is too many calories in the diet. Most individuals would be far better off, nutritionally, if they could reduce their dietary fat intake to a value of about 30 to 35 percent of total caloric intake. Table 5 illustrates the proportion of fat (by calories) in some popular foods.

From the standpoint of the runner, a meal that is high in fat is not recommended just prior to exercise. Fat has been shown to slow down digestion and gastric emptying and may remain in the gastrointestinal tract for as long as 12 hours. Even though fat supplies a large portion of energy during a long-distance run, it can be derived from the large amount of fat stored in the adipose cells (fat cells) of the body and does not have to come from dietary sources.

Proteins

Proteins are vital for life since they are the building blocks required to make body tissues for new growth and replacement of worn-out cells. Each person must consume a certain amount of protein each day in order to meet the needs of tissue synthesis. The recommended daily dietary allowance (RDA) for protein in the United States (values are set by the National Research Council) for adults is 0.8 grams per kilogram of body weight. For example, a 70 kilogram male (154 pounds) requires 56 grams of protein per day. Table 6 lists some typical foods and the amount of protein (in grams) present in each.

Most athletes are concerned about not getting enough protein. Is this a valid concern? Scientific studies have shown that protein requirements for athletes are similar to those of more sedentary people, when adjusted to the greater caloric intake of the athlete. One reason for this may be that the United States RDA values are typically set generously high. Basically, there is a safety factor built into all the RDA figures. In addition, it is quite common for the average American to consume considerably more protein, approaching 1.2 to 1.5 grams per kilogram of body weight. It is apparent that protein deficiency is not a problem in this country.

One of the latest dietary fads, one that has tempted both athletes as well as nonathletes, is the promotion of consuming individual amino acids, such as

TABLE 5. Total Caloric Value and Proportion of Fat of Some Typical Food Items. Values are Without Anything Added to Foods.

Food or Beverage	*Weight or Measure*	*Total Calories*	*% of Calories from Fat*
Milk (Whole)	1 cup	160	51
Milk (Lowfat)	1 cup	145	31
Cheddar Cheese	1 oz.	115	70
Cottage Cheese	1 cup	260	35
Swiss Cheese	1 oz.	105	69
Yoghurt (Skim milk)	1 cup	125	29
Ice Cream	1 cup	255	49
Eggs (Whole)	1	80	68
Bacon	2 slices	90	80
Hamburger (Reg.)	3 oz.	245	62
Steak (Sirloin)	3 oz.	330	74
Steak (Round)	3 oz.	220	53
Chicken	3 oz.	115	23
Pork Chop	2.3 oz.	260	73
Frankfurter	1	170	79
Peanuts	1 cup	840	77
Bread (Whole wheat)	1 slice	65	14
Pie (Apple)	1 sector	350	39
Butter	1 pat	35	100
Fast Foods			
Burger King Whopper	1	606	48
French Fries	1 serving	214	42
Vanilla Shake	1	332	30
McDonald's Big Mac	1	541	52

tryptophan, among others. There are so many claims for these nutrient supplements that it would be difficult to cover them all in a paragraph. Some of the claims include improvement in reaction and movement time, an improvement in either intelligence or other cerebral activities, and a decrease in appetite. There has been no scientific documentation for any of the claims being made for this nutritional supplement. Amino acids are the building blocks of protein molecules, and are consumed in more than sufficient quantities with total protein

TABLE 6. Caloric Value and Protein of Some Typical Food Items.

Note that foods marked with an asterisk are considered incomplete proteins and should be combined with other incomplete proteins or with complete protein foods.

Food or Beverage	*Weight or Measure*	*Total Calories*	*Grams of Proteins*
Milk (Whole)	1 cup	160	9
Cheddar Cheese	1 oz.	115	7
Cottage Cheese	1 cup	260	33
Ice Cream	1 cup	255	6
Eggs (Whole)	1	80	6
Hamburger (Regular)	3 oz.	245	21
Steak (Sirloin)	3 oz.	330	20
Chicken	3 oz.	115	20
Salmon (Pink)	3 oz.	120	17
Shrimp	3 oz.	100	21
Tuna	3 oz.	170	24
Beans (Red kidney)*	1 cup	230	15
Peanuts*	1 cup	840	37
Beans (Lima)*	1 cup	190	13
Bread (Whole wheat)*	1 slice	65	3
Macaroni*	1 cup	190	6
Pizza (Cheese)	1 slice	185	7
Rice*	1 cup	225	4
Peanut Butter*	1 tbsp.	95	4
Potatoes*	1	90	3
Spinach*	1 cup	40	5
Corn*	1 ear	70	3
Broccoli*	1 stalk	45	6
Fast Foods			
Burger King Whopper	1	606	29
McDonald's Big Mac	1	541	26
Kentucky Fried Chicken	3 pieces	653	53
Taco Bell Burrito Supreme	1	457	21

ingestion. Since the American diet supplies so much protein, it makes no sense to consume additional quantities of these substances.

Vitamins and Minerals

Perhaps the most overused nutritional supplements by athletes are vitamins and minerals. Many people feel that these substances, especially vitamins, will give added pep and vitality. Television advertisements often refer to conditions such as "tired blood," and encourage the use of substances such as Geritol (iron supplement). Athletes are particularly vulnerable to claims of increased energy or vitality from food supplements. After running 10 or 15 miles, you may be completely fatigued. If you were promised relief from that fatigue by taking a vitamin, you would probably jump at the opportunity. It is difficult to ignore these claims and promises without some basic knowledge in nutrition.

What are vitamins and minerals? A *vitamin* is an organic (contains carbon) compound needed for growth, maintenance, and regulation of metabolic processes. Deficiency of any vitamin will result in disease (i.e., thiamine (B1 = Beriberi) or a pathological condition (vitamin A (Retinol) = night blindness). Minerals are inorganic substances that are used as structural components (i.e., calcium and phosphorus in bone) and as regulators of body processes (i.e., magnesium in metabolism). An entire book could be written about the function of each specific vitamin and mineral needed by the body. However, it should be sufficient to state here that there is no scientific evidence to indicate that athletes require greater amounts of these nutrients.

In making this statement, the following assumptions must be made:

1. The athlete consumes a well-balanced diet that includes food from all four basic food groups.
2. The athlete consumes a greater amount of calories, which represents his or her greater caloric expenditure. These extra calories are derived from eating good, nutritious foods (not "junk" foods).

Well-controlled scientific studies indicate that supplementation with vitamins E, C, and B complex as well as the magical Pangamic Acid ("B-15"), do not result in improved physical performance (Watt, Romet, McFarlane, McGuey, Allen, & Goode, 1974; Lawrence, Bower, Riehl, & Smith, 1975; Buskirk, 1977; Girandola, Wiswell, & Bulbulian, 1980). The best advice would be to not spend money on nutritional supplements and spend the money on good quality foods. Enjoy the food and the pleasures of eating.

Electrolytes

Every long-distance runner is concerned about maintaining normal electrolyte balance. During most long-distance runs, some form of fluid supplement is available. Commercial solutions such as Gatorade ®, E.R.G. ®, and Quick

Kick ® are on the market and among the many claims made are that electrolytes are replenished. What are electrolytes? They are substances whose water solutions conduct electric current as a result of ionization or dissociation. Electrolytes in human fluids are calcium, phosphate, magnesium, sodium, potassium, chloride, and sulfate. The runner, of course, is concerned that sweat loss may cause depletion of one or more of these electrolytes. This depletion may, in turn, cause severe muscle cramping, as well as other problems. Experimental evidence does not support the claim that electrolyte depletion is a common problem during long-distance running. The only mineral that may decrease somewhat is potassium (K) and the recommendation is that the runner eat some high-potassium foods prior to the race (such as tomatoes, bananas, and citrus fruits). In very long-distance running, the best solution is to drink a cold (40° F) hypotonic (very dilute) glucose solution.

Water

Most individuals do not even consider water when discussing nutrition and performance. However, the runner must be particularly concerned with fluid balance. Water is lost through the lungs, urine, feces, and sweat. Ingested fluid is obtained from drinking and eating. The important thing to remember is that during a long run it is very easy to lose 2 to 3 quarts of water. Therefore, during and after the run, you must drink enough to make up for this fluid deficit. Severe dehydration, which is not uncommon in distance runners, may lead to heat prostration and heat stroke. You should not be afraid to drink plenty of liquid before, during, and after the exercise. The thirst mechanism in a human is not very finely tuned; thus your conscious desire to drink is not set for the amount lost. During a marathon run, you may only replace 10 percent of the water that is lost as sweat, even though you ingest water at all of the aid stations. Liquid ingestion should be done before, during, and after the run. Even though you do not feel thirsty, you should attempt to get fluid ingested, especially during the run.

What and When to Eat or Drink Before Running

Athletes often have very bizarre eating habits, especially just prior to an athletic event. Some prefer not to eat, others love steaks, and still others may opt for liquid meals. There is no ideal meal for everyone; it becomes a matter of preference. However, certain guidelines should be kept in mind. Studies show that an individual can eat a liquid or solid meal (of about 1000 calories) as late as 30 minutes prior to running without experiencing any gastrointestinal disturbances. It should be mentioned that this meal was made up of approximately 30 percent fat. It is possible that a meal of different composition (greater fat?) would have a more negative effect.

As mentioned earlier, pre-exercise meals should be higher in CHO and lower in fat. In addition, items such as beans, cabbage, and other gas-producing foods should be eliminated. High fiber foods (i.e., vegetables) should not be overemphasized. Finally, new or "exotic" foods should not be consumed as a pre-exercise meal; you should stay with menu items that you are accustomed to.

A study by Ivy, Costill, Fink, and Lower (1979) indicates that caffeine ingestion may be helpful in endurance exercise. However, you should be aware of the problems associated with caffeine ingestion, prior to consuming large amounts. Caffeine is a potent diuretic which causes an increase in urine loss and accentuates the dehydration caused by sweating. In addition, caffeine is known to increase acid secretion in the stomach and has been implicated in ulcer development in susceptible individuals. Coffee (which has a very high level of caffeine) may be of some benefit but the effects are certainly not very great, and intake should be tempered against long-term health effects.

Summary

An understanding of proper nutritional intake is very important for anyone undertaking a vigorous exercise program. You expend calories during both rest and exercise. That expenditure must be balanced by an adequate caloric intake or weight loss will result. Weight changes that occur after exercise are almost always due to hydration changes. In addition to body weight changes that occur during exercise, body composition alterations occur. These are usually seen as a reduction in percentage of body fat and an increase in lean body mass.

An adequate diet for a long-distance runner requires sufficient calories to meet expenditure, CHO ingestion amounting to 50 to 60 percent of total calories. A proper selection of items from the four basic food groups is expected to supply adequate protein, vitamins, and minerals for an active individual.

Review

1. Caloric balance is determined by comparing caloric intake to caloric expenditure.
2. In order to lose one pound of weight, you must create a deficit of 3500 calories.

3. The caloric equivalent of running is measured at about 100 calories per mile.
4. Total body water accounts for approximately 60 percent of body weight and usually accounts for the dramatic changes in body weight observed after exercise.
5. An average male and female possess 15 and 25 percent body fat, respectively. However, very lean distance runners of both sexes are much lower in body fat.
6. Extreme leanness in females may coincide with problems with menstrual function.
7. CHO loading is a means of increasing the glycogen level in the muscle cells and thereby improving endurance performance.
8. Protein requirement for a runner should amount to no more than 1 gram per kilogram of body weight.
9. The benefits of supplementing a good diet with vitamin-mineral supplements, for sedentary people or runners, are not substantiated by scientific evidence.
10. Water is the substance that must be ingested during and after long-distance running, especially in warm climates.
11. Electrolyte replacement during exercise has not been found to be necessary.

CHAPTER 8

Influence of Environmental Conditions on Running

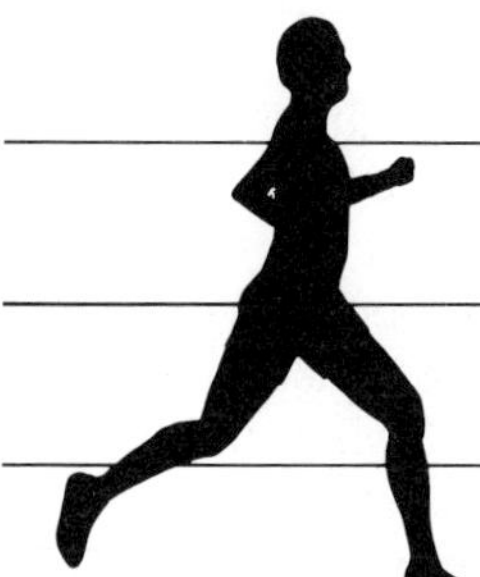

If you run outdoors every day of the year, you are subjected to various environmental conditions that vary depending on geographical location. Extreme heat and cold, high and low humidity, and wind and smog are among the conditions that runners must learn to cope with. Some of these environmental conditions may simply cause mild discomfort, while others may be extremely dangerous to exercise in.

Heat

When the ambient temperature is high, running long distances can be extremely difficult. A basic understanding of thermal balance in humans is essential for those who expect to exercise under these conditions. Humans are classified as *homeotherms*; that is, they maintain a relatively constant internal or core temperature (98.6 degrees F). The internal heat is produced by normal cellular metabolism (described in Chapter 2) and varies depending on the amount of fuel being oxidized. During exercise, when large amounts of fuel are being catabolized, internal heat increases tremendously. For example, heat production can range from 90 calories per hour at rest to as much as 1200 calories per hour during heavy exercise. The ability to dissipate this heat is critical to the athlete. During very heavy exercise, the heat produced could theoretically increase body temperature from 98.6 degrees F to about 140 degrees F if excess heat were not dissipated. Of course, the upper limit for internal temperature is only about 107 to 108 degrees F, so the theoretical individual would be long gone.

Methods by which the human body dissipates heat are generally well known. They include the following.

Radiation

Radiation is the transfer of heat or energy to or from the environment to the surface of the body in the form of electromagnetic waves. Radiative heat gain or loss (from the body, to or from the environment) depends primarily on ambient temperature. Thus, if the ambient temperature is over 95 degrees F, the individual will gain some heat. In addition to the temperature gradient, there is also the radiant energy absorption from the sun that is magnified when there is no cloud cover. This is called *infrared heat gain*. If a thermometer is placed in the sun on a warm cloudless day, the sun (infrared temperature) temperature may exceed shade temperature by almost 20 degrees F. This is why overcast days are more comfortable for the long-distance runner when ambient temperature is high.

Convection

Convection is the heat exchange between an object and the currents of gas or liquid that flow past the object. Essentially, the greater the wind speed, the greater the heat loss. On a hot day a slight wind can be very comforting to a runner.

Perspiration

Perspiration is the heat loss that occurs through the action of sweat glands. *Evaporative heat loss* is defined as the heat required to change water from liquid to the vapor state. This means that, in order for heat loss to occur, sweat must evaporate from the skin. To get an idea of how this works, try putting some alcohol on your skin; it will feel very cool. The cooling sensation is caused by the rapid evaporation of the alcohol.

Heat Balance

There are some important implications concerning heat balance that you should understand. First, the ability to lose heat by sweating is perhaps the most important method of maintaining heat balance during heavy exercise. However, sweat does not evaporate readily when the air is already saturated with water. Thus, when the relative humidity is above 90 percent, evaporative cooling is detrimentally affected.

The second important factor concerns the runner's clothing. It is quite fashionable to wear jogging suits and other clothing when running. Whether these items are worn as a fad or in the belief that they are really necessary for running well is known only to the specific person. Clothing worn over the trunk and legs definitely impairs evaporation of sweat. Therefore, the ideal situation is to wear as little as possible—shorts and shirt (women). In addition, the type of material worn is important. Nylon and other synthetic fibers oppose water vapor passage and thus are not recommended. Cotton is the ideal material for clothing to be worn in the heat since it is relatively light and presents no great barrier to evaporation. Small holes in the clothing are also helpful. A new synthetic material, polypropylene, also appears to be pervious to water (sweat).

You should also be aware of a potentially dangerous situation that occurs when you wear a plastic or rubber suit during running. Typically, these suits are worn by individuals who are attempting to lose weight. When these suits are removed after a workout, invariably they are filled with water (sweat), and sure enough the wearer has lost weight (fluid loss). However, the fluid that is so readily visible after the suit is removed is actually sweat that has not evaporated. Wearing plastic or rubber material (or any other material that is impervious to moisture) prevents evaporative cooling and also impairs radiative heat loss, to some degree. If you wore this type of clothing on a very warm day and ran far enough, it is very likely that you would collapse from heat prostration or heat stroke.

Heat and Humidity

When you run for long distances, the major environmental problem that you will face is a high ambient temperature coupled with high humidity. From a geographical standpoint, these are common summer conditions on the eastern seaboard and along the Gulf coast. While running, your body dissipates heat primarily by radiation and perspiration. If the ambient temperature is high, as well as relative humidity, the body cannot dissipate heat readily. Continued running simply overloads the body's attempts at heat dissipation and serious consequences could ensue. Those that appear to be most sensitive to heat overloads include the elderly, children, the obese, and the unconditioned individual, in general. During a 14-kilometer road race in Australia several years ago, twenty-nine runners collapsed from heat stress, and the temperature was a relatively mild 50 degrees F!

Symptoms of Heat Injury

Since heat injuries can occur so frequently in distance running, you should be aware of the warning signs of impending collapse. These symptoms include some or all of the following: headache, nausea, disorientation, faintness, visual disturbances, fatigue, diarrhea, cramps, weak rapid pulse, pallor, pale cold skin, and cessation of sweating. If body temperature is measured in the affected individual it may read as high as 106 degrees F. Immediate treatment for heat injury aims at trying to lower body temperature. The subject should rest supine, preferably in the shade. Ice packs and/or alcohol rubs should be applied. If the victim is conscious, liquid should be given and perhaps a mild stimulant, such as cold tea.

Precautions

Ideally, you should never get into an environmental situation (high temperature and humidity) where heat problems are likely to occur. However, if you are entered in a race under these conditions, certain adjustments should be made. You should drink about 400 to 500 ml (13 to 17 ounces) of fluid before starting and then about 100 ml every 2 to 3 miles (assuming it is available). You should not "push" yourself extremely hard during the race. Under these ambient conditions, your pace should be slower than normal and, if symptoms of heat stress should occur, the pace should be slowed even more, perhaps to a walk. Often, heat injuries can result in disorientation which prevents you from realizing that you may be in serious trouble. A classic case of heat-related injury was witnessed by millions of viewers on television during the finish of the women's marathon at the 1984 Olympics. One of the women competitors literally staggered across the finish line in the Los Angeles Coliseum. Fortunately for this runner, the medical outcome was quite favorable.

Individual Differences in Heat Tolerance

The ability to tolerate heat varies from person to person. A thin person has a larger surface area to weight ratio, as compared to a squat, overweight individual. Therefore, radiative heat loss is greater for the thin runner. The more subcutaneous fat an individual possesses, the more difficult it is to dissipate heat. Sweat rate also displays large individual differences, with heat-acclimatized individuals possessing a much greater ability to sweat.

There are approximately two million sweat glands in the skin of an average person. The more you have, the better it is, since the ability to sweat is definitely an advantage when running in the heat. Although there are some differences of opinion, it appears that female athletes perspire at the same rate as their male counterparts. Young children and older individuals (over 50 years) appear to tolerate the heat less well than young adults. For young children, heat intolerance appears to be related primarily to their immature cardiovascular system. (With prolonged sweating, plasma volume decreases, lowering total blood volume. This puts an added strain on the cardiovascular system, since it is this parameter that helps in heat dissipation.) In the older adult, heat intolerance is due to an inadequate sweating response and a decrease in cardiovascular fitness. Therefore, children and older adults should be scrutinized more closely during long-distance running in hot environments.

Cold

During the winter season throughout most of the United States, temperatures typically drop to freezing (32 degrees F) and below. For the runner who wishes to continue his or her training outdoors, it is simply one more obstacle to overcome. In reality, long-distance running when the ambient temperature is low is much less of a hazard to the runner than when the temperature is high. The incidence of hypothermia (low body temperature) in runners is far less frequent than hyperthermia (high body temperature). However, some problems could develop and, therefore, everyone should be aware of the physiological adaptations to a cold environment.

The problem of a hot environment involves the body's inability to dissipate heat. In a cold environment, the dilemma is in trying to retain heat or, more accurately, to maintain core temperature. When an individual is exposed to cold, his or her body essentially shuts down blood flow to the periphery (skin and extremities). Unless you get into a life or death situation (i.e., becominig stranded or lost in bitter cold), core temperature will usually be maintained.

Retaining Heat

While running in the cold, the main concern should be in trying to protect exposed areas and extremities (i.e., face, head, hands, and feet). Wearing extra socks, mittens or gloves, ski mask, and hat should be sufficient. You should also be aware of the fact that body heat will dissipate rapidly from any area of the body that is not protected by clothing. For example, large amounts of body heat will be lost through your scalp if your head is not protected and, therefore, you will definitely feel cold. Clothing is our basic means of protection against ambient cold temperature. Radiative heat loss is prevented by the insulating capabilities of clothing.

The key to being comfortable in a cold environment involves wearing proper materials and the correct amount of them. For instance, cotton, which is recommended for high temperatures because of its light weight and porosity, offers little protection from cold. Wool is generally the best fabric to wear in the cold since it absorbs moisture (sweat) and offers good insulation. A good combination would be cotton, close to the skin, and wool over that. If there is any wind, a nylon or Gore-tex ® parka over the wool would also help. Many novice runners make the mistake of wearing too much clothing. You should remember that while running body heat increases dramatically. The ambient temperature that would normally feel so uncomfortable on first exposure becomes quite bearable after you "warm up."

Windchill

Just as the combination of heat and humidity can make running in the summer unbearable, a combination of cold and wind can take their toll in the winter months. The *effective temperature* is a common description of ambient conditions in the winter. Essentially, it is a table that gives a perceived temperature, based on ambient temperature, humidity, and wind velocity. It is also referred to as the *windchill factor*. For example, an ambient temperature of 0 degrees F with a wind velocity of 10 MPH gives an effective temperature of −40 degrees F! The "windchill" description for this condition states "exposed flesh freezes, travel disagreeable." Clearly these are not good running conditions. You should also note that running at 8 MPH directly into a 5 MPH headwind is equivalent to a 13 MPH headwind!

Breathing Discomfort

Another cold-related problem runners are concerned with is that of breathing very cold air. Some runners feel that this cold air can be damaging to the lungs. Actually, this is not a valid concern since the air is essentially warmed to body temperature before it reaches the alveoli. However, because the air is cold and dry, it causes dryness and some constriction of the upper airways. This can cause some breathing discomfort, especially in hypersensitive individuals. People with asthma often have difficulty during exercise while breathing cold, dry air.

Altitude

There may be instances when you visit an area that is well above sea level. Running (or any other form of physical work) at altitude presents some problems if you are unacclimatized. The higher the altitude, the lower number of oxygen molecules in the air. This translates into fewer oxygen molecules in the blood and a decrease in aerobic exercise performance. It has been estimated that for every 1000 feet you ascend above 5000 feet, there is a 3 percent reduction in maximal oxygen consumption. Thus, you would expect poorer endurance performance at altitude.

If you have the opportunity to run at altitude you should keep in mind that exercise intensity will feel much higher than at sea level. That is, since the maximal capacity is decreased, any submaximal training load will be concomitantly higher at altitude, as compared to sea level. There is really no danger in running at low to moderate altitudes. You simply must take into consideration that you should run at a slower pace (and perhaps a shorter distance) than you would if you were at sea level.

If you remain at altitude for several weeks you will acclimatize (adapt physiologically) to the higher elevation. This adaptation is seen as an increase in the number of red blood cells and the amount of hemoglobin in the blood. This change allows for greater oxygen-carrying capacity of the blood. Thus, you will be able to tolerate the altitude more readily since maximal capacity will be elevated.

Air Pollution

In most of our urban environments there is a substantial level of air pollution caused by emissions from automobiles, factories, and refineries, among others. From the standpoint of the runner who lives in this type of environment and must breathe this polluted air, what are the short- and long-term consequences? Many runners (and other athletes as well) are so concerned with the pollution that they fear more harm than good will come from exercising under these adverse conditions. Some of these fears may be well-founded.

The type of pollutant indigenous to an area depends on the type of emission. For example, in southern California, automobile exhaust is the major emission, which results in large amounts of carbon monoxide, ozone, and nitrogen oxides. In the highly industrial East coast cities, the major pollutants are carbon monoxide and sulfur oxides (from burning coal).

Many of these terms may sound rather imposing to someone who wishes to preserve the integrity of his or her lungs. Most of the evidence to date has not implicated air pollution, at currently appearing levels, as a major health problem. Certainly some individuals—those with existing pulmonaray dysfunction or allergies—are much more susceptible to the effects of air pollution. The recent Olympic Games (1984) that were held in Los Angeles, California, were a testimonial to the fact that air pollution cannot be considered a major problem for athletic performance, or short-term health. However, it should also be mentioned that there were no episodes of very high levels of air pollution (ozone) during the period of the games.

The long-term effects of exercising in a moderately polluted environment have not been determined as yet. The best suggestion that could be made to you if you live in this kind of environment, would simply be to avoid exercise during peak levels of pollution, or near areas where there are sure to be high levels. For example, during the summer in the southern California area, ozone levels vary based on time of day. Ozone levels usually peak between 12 noon and 4 P.M. Therefore, the best time to run is early morning or late at night (on most days). Also you should avoid running near a major thoroughfare or any area of high traffic congestion. It was found that runners exercising in New York City near the East River Drive, a high traffic area, had a higher level of carbon monoxide in their blood than those simply walking in this area (but not exercising) and also compared to runners in other, less congested areas of the city.

Running is so beneficial to many, from both a physiological as well as a psychological standpoint, that it would be foolish to give up this recreational activity because you live in a crowded city. The benefits of running will probably make up for any negative effects that breathing in some of the various pollutants would cause. However, as stated earlier, running should be done during times of the day, or in areas of the city, that are relatively clean.

Summary

The environmental conditions that you must run in vary with the seasons of the year as well as with geographical location. During summer months, you must be able to tolerate high ambient temperatures and often high humidity as well. During the winter months, depending on where you live, you must be able to withstand cold, wind, rain, and snow. If you travel to an area where the altitude is greater than 5000 feet, you must understand the problems encountered there. Finally, in most urban settings, the problem of air pollution is ever present.

Review

1. The human body dissipates heat primarily by radiation, convection, and perspiration. The method depends on the environmental conditions.
2. The combination of high ambient temperature and relative humidity make for very difficult conditions for long-distance running.
3. The ability to tolerate heat during running depends on body dimensions, age, and the number of active sweat glands.
4. Although hypothermia during running is much less frequent than hyperthermia, you should still be aware of conditions that might cause the problem.

5. A combination of low ambient temperature, wind, and wet clothing are all conducive to causing a drop in body temperature.
6. Because of the decrease in oxygen molecules at altitude, maximal oxygen consumption decreases in almost direct proportion to the elevation.
7. Acclimatization to altitude occurs after several weeks of exposure and is manifested as an increase in red blood cells.
8. Air pollution is a very real hazard for runners in certain urban areas. The major pollutants include ozone, carbon monoxide, and sulfur oxides.

CHAPTER 9
Stretching and Warm-Up

Stretching and warm-up exercises are extremely important to the runner who wishes to remain injury-free and to maximize performance while training and racing. It is important to understand the physiological reasons for stretching and warm-up and then to incorporate a program into your daily activities.

Stretching and Flexibility

While the necessity to stretch muscles prior to and following activities such as sprinting (and all sports that require participants to sprint) is unquestioned, the need to stretch prior to distance running is an arguable point. However, the general rule in any program of physical activity that involves heavy muscle activity is to combine strengthening and stretching activities. For many individuals, a program of proper stretching movements helps prevent many of the ailments that accompany a running program. It should be emphasized that when the term *stretching* is applied, it is applied to the muscle. In other words, the goal is to stretch the muscle rather than the joint between two muscles.

Static and Dynamic Stretching

Stretching before and after running may be necessary for many individuals in order to prevent injury to the muscles, tendons, and ligaments during strong muscular contractions. In some individuals who have a limited range of motion, a program of stretching will help improve this range and allow the individual to run more smoothly and efficiently. There are basically two types of stretching—static and dynamic. A static stretch involves applying a consistent force toward a long slow holding of a position at the limit of your muscle length. This stretch is usually held for a 30-second to 2-minute period. In contrast, the dynamic (also called ballistic stretch) stretch requires you to bounce in and out of certain positions, usually in a series of rapid movements. This type of stretch fires muscle spindles for a "stretch" reflex contraction of the muscles that you are attempting to stretch. Therefore, this type of stretch is contraindicated.

Warm-Up and Warm-Down

The importance of warming up before running should also be understood. Warm-up serves to increase muscle temperature in order for the muscles to perform optimally. (Stretching exercises do *not* increase muscle temperature.) The warming up of the muscles will also allow you to reach the "steady-state" faster. In running, the warm-up usually consists of jogging at a moderate pace for a mile. If you expect to be in a competitive race where the pace will be reasonably fast (i.e., a 10 kilometer race in under 40 minutes), a few sprints all out and some sprints with very high knee lifts are recommended.

Warm-up is extremely important for the middle-aged individual. Some middle-aged men display abnormal EKG patterns (ischemic response) when they begin exercising without prior warm-up. However, the amount of prior warm-up should be determined by the eventual workout or race. For example, the individuals who displayed abnormal EKGs were placed on a treadmill and requested to jog at a fairly rapid pace, almost immediately (Barnard, Gardner, Diaco, Macalpin, & Kattus, 1973). If you begin your workout by jogging slowly, a warm-up may not be necessary. If you are about to go on a very long run (10 miles or more) it would not be very wise to waste energy by warming up. This assumes that you are not in competition and, therefore, the initial pace at the beginning of the race is unimportant. Stretching is recommended for everyone; warming-up is recommended only for certain specific situations and individuals.

The concept of warm-down is another activity that is not well understood by athletes or coaches. Running is a large muscle activity that involves the leg muscles, such as the quadriceps, gastrocnemius, and hamstrings, among others. While the muscles are active during running, a large amount of blood is being directed to the leg muscles. As the muscles contract they are actually helping "push" the venous blood back up toward the heart. This is called the *accessory muscle pump*. At the end of the run, even if you stop completely, a large amount of blood is still directed toward your leg muscles (the recovery process). If you are standing upright, the blood being directed to your leg muscles must "fight" gravity, without the aid of contracting leg muscles, to get back to the heart muscle. Often, if you stop an activity such as running or bicycling, and stand erect there may be blood pooling in your legs and you may get somewhat lightheaded as there is a deficiency of blood to the central nervous system. The reason for warm-down (or cool-down) is to maintain the accessory muscle pump action until the need for blood in the lower extremities decreases. This should not take more than several minutes. Good warm-down exercises include jogging lightly or walking quickly.

Stretching: A Practical Approach

Figures 37 through 44 depict a series of stretching exercises that are recommended for most individuals in order to help maintain an injury-free running program. While increasing the flexibility of the musculature will not *ensure*

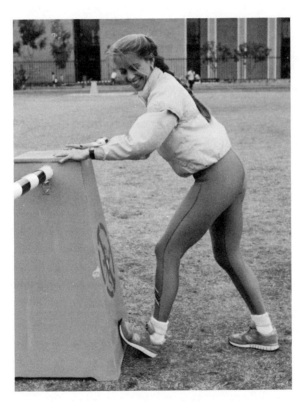

FIGURE 37. Stretching of the gastrocnemius and soleus muscles.

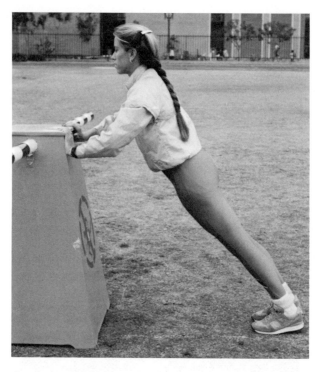

FIGURE 38. Another method of stretching the gastrocnemius and soleus muscles.

injury prevention, the evidence indicates that it may be beneficial. It should be pointed out, however, that everyone is constructed a little differently. Flexibility varies markedly from person to person. Some individuals have an enormous range of motion, while others are extremely "tight." In recommending these exercises, it should be emphasized that you perform them to your specific limitations.

Lower leg. Figures 37 and 38 demonstrate exercises that can be utilized to stretch the muscles that are typically called the *calf* (gastrocnemius and soleus) muscle. These stretches are very important since Achilles tendonitis is a very common injury in runners and these movements will help alleviate some of the problem. Both movements should be done for at least 2 minutes each.

Front, lower leg. Figure 39 illustrates an excellent exercise for the proper stretching of the anterior (front) muscles of the lower leg. The foot is grasped with the hand on same side and pulled upwards and backwards. This exercise also stretches the large muscle of the thigh (quadriceps).

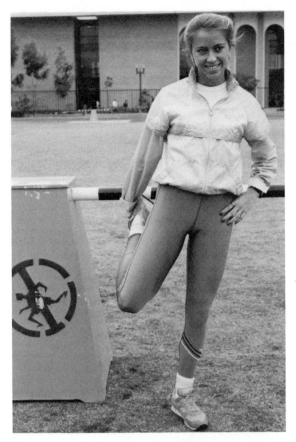

FIGURE 39. Stretching the muscles of the front of the lower leg and the quadriceps muscle (thigh).

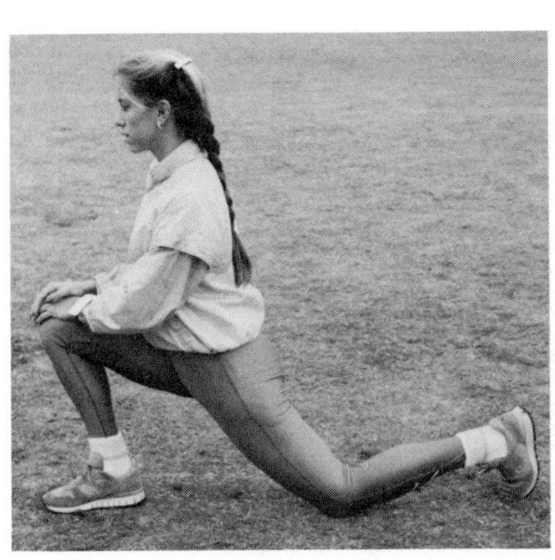

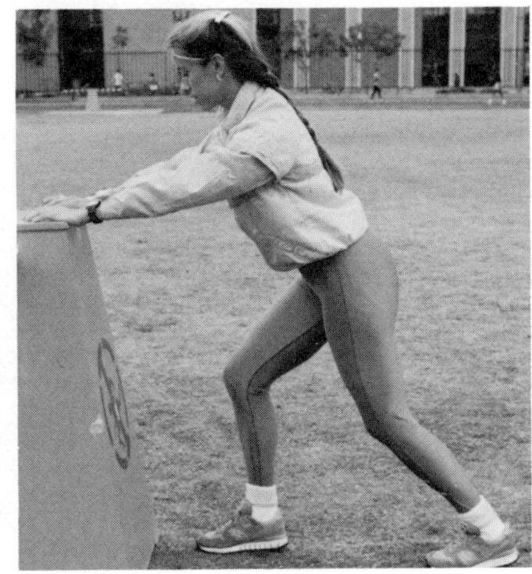

FIGURE 40. Stretching the quadriceps muscle.

Front, upper leg. Figures 40 and 41 demonstrate stretching exercises that can be used to stretch the large upper thigh muscle—the quadriceps femoris. This muscle extends over the knee joint and these exercises also help somewhat for this joint. The movement in Figure 41 can also double as a "calf" stretcher.

Front, upper leg and trunk. Figure 42 demonstrates an exercise that stretches both the quadriceps muscle as well as the abdominal muscle. Often the muscles of the trunk, both front and back, become tight as a result of running a great deal. Although the flexibility of the upper trunk is usually not a problem, it is still recommended that some attention be given to the musculature in this area.

Back, upper leg. No stretching program would be complete without some exercises designed to increase the flexibility of the large muscles located at the

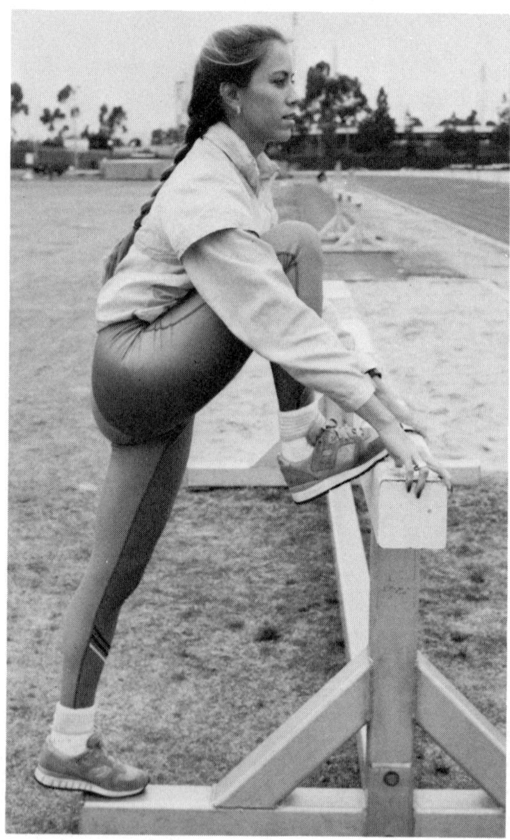

FIGURE 41. Stretching the quadriceps, gastrocnemius, and soleus muscles.

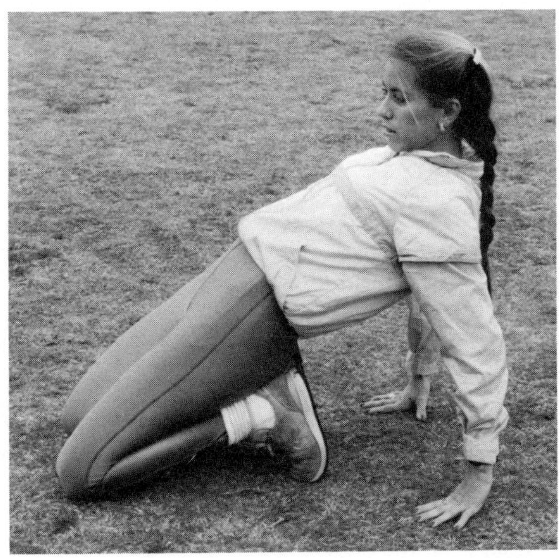

FIGURE 42. Stretching the quadriceps and abdominal musculature of the anterior trunk.

back of the upper thigh. These muscles are collectively called the *hamstrings.* Although this is a greater problem area for sprinters (muscle pulls are very common), injuries to this muscle also occur in distance runners. Part of the problem stems from the fact that this muscle is termed a *flexor* (decreases the angle of a joint) and these muscles are more susceptible to decreased flexibility. Another problem stems from the fact that the opposite-acting muscle, the quadriceps, is usually much stronger. Figure 43 shows classic exercises designed to stretch the hamstrings.

Lower back. Figure 44 demonstrates an exercise that can be utilized to improve the flexibility of the lower back. The lower back is a problem area for many runners, although not necessarily due to lack of flexibility. Nonetheless, it is recommended that, in addition to stretching of the abdominal area, you do the same for your back.

A vigorous and regular program of proper stretching exercises may prevent or alleviate muscular injuries that are often associated with long-distance running. Even though you may feel no need to improve flexibility, it is a well-known fact that lack of flexibility is a problem associated with aging. A program of stretching, begun at a relatively early age, may help prevent some of problems many aged individuals face, in terms of ambulation.

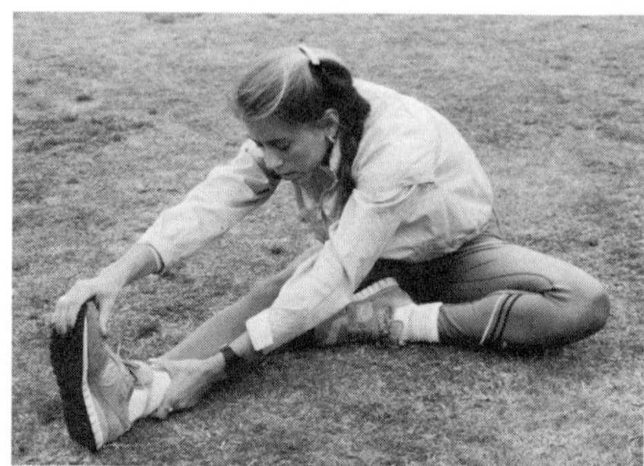

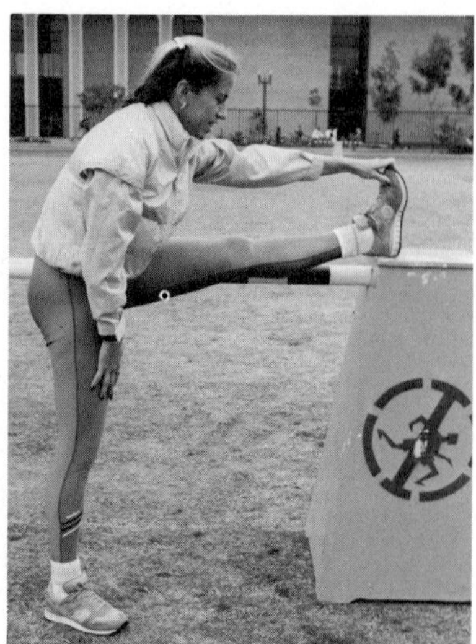

FIGURE 43. Stretching the hamstring muscle group.

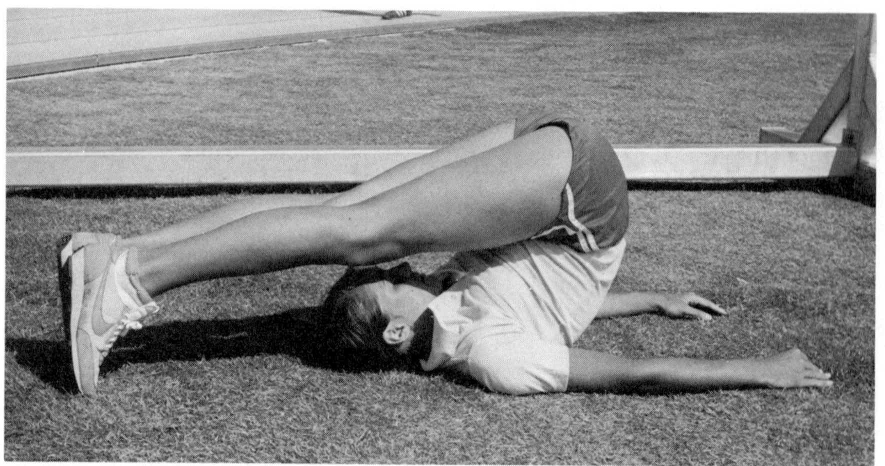

FIGURE 44. Stretching the lower back is always a good idea for long-distance runners.

Summary

A regular program of muscle stretching and warm-up is highly recommended for a runner. Warming up prior to running involves performing dynamic exercises to elevate muscle temperature. Warm-down is also important following the completion of a long run. A series of stretching exercises are presented. Ideally, these exercises should be performed prior to, and following, any run to help minimize the incidence of muscle injuries.

Review

1. Warming up prior to any subsequent exercise involves performing activities that will elevate muscle temperature.
2. Warm-down (or cool-down) following running is necessary to prevent blood pooling in the lower extremities.
3. Static stretching, performed prior to and following a run, is an important measure to help prevent muscle injuries.
4. A series of photographs depicts some of the more popular stretching exercises that you should incorporate into a regular program.

APPENDIX Personal Running Log

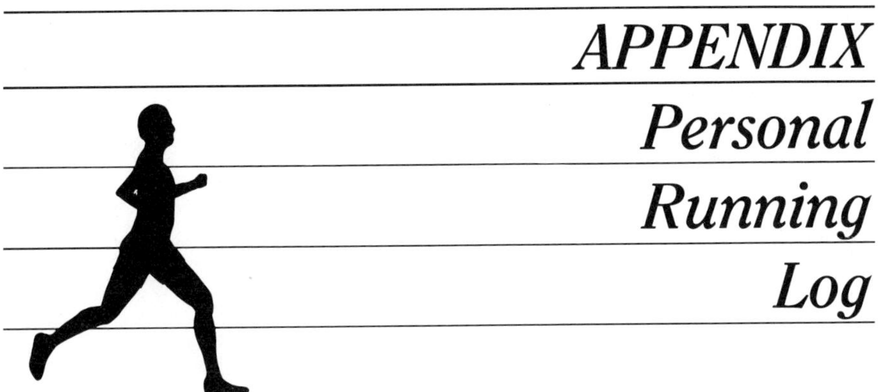

The following tables represent a suggested method of maintaining a running "diary." If you are just starting a running program, it is extremely valuable in that it allows you to visualize the progress you have made. Motivation plays a major part in running, and there is nothing more motivating than visualizing your progress, in either tabular or graphic format. Included are spaces for the distance covered (i.e., 1 mile, 10 km, etc.), total elapsed time, climatic conditions (weather), type of terrain (i.e, hills, trails, track), resting and post-exercise heart rate, and subjective feelings. Monitoring your heart rate before and after running will give you a good progress report on physiological adaptation to the training program. Regarding the space for subjective feelings, you can express how you felt during and after the run. For example, you may have felt "very tired" or had a "pain in the side," or perhaps you "felt great." It may be of interest to look back on the diary after you have been running for a long period of time and see how you have adapted in terms of physiological as well as psychological effects. Try to be meticulous about the running log, just as you should be with your running program.

Personal Running Log

Day	Climatic Condition	Running Terrain	Distance Covered	Elapsed Time	Heart Rate		Subjective Feelings
					Resting	Post-Exercise	
Monday							
Tuesday							
Wednesday							
Thursday							
Friday							
Saturday							
Sunday							

Personal Running Log

Day	Climatic Condition	Running Terrain	Distance Covered	Elapsed Time	Heart Rate		Subjective Feelings
					Resting	Post-Exercise	
Monday							
Tuesday							
Wednesday							
Thursday							
Friday							
Saturday							
Sunday							

Personal Running Log

Day	Climatic Condition	Running Terrain	Distance Covered	Elapsed Time	Heart Rate		Subjective Feelings
					Resting	Post-Exercise	
Monday							
Tuesday							
Wednesday							
Thursday							
Friday							
Saturday							
Sunday							

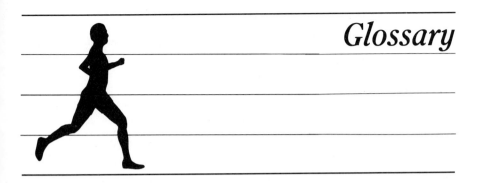

Glossary

Acclimatization Physiological adaptation to continued exposure to a different environment.

Achilles tendon Fibrous connective tissue at the lower end of the gastrocnemius muscle.

Adenosine triphosphate (ATP) The chemical molecule in the body most available for energy release.

Adipose cell A specialized cell in the body that stores fat.

Aerobic cycle Energy production when oxygen is available.

Alveoli Small air cells of the lungs, through which gas exchange occurs.

Ambience Surrounding environmental conditions.

Amenorrhea Absence or suppression of menstruation.

Anaerobic cycle Energy production without oxygen.

Anaerobic threshold The exercise intensity, relative to the individual, that anaerobic energy production predominates.

Bicycle ergometer Stationary bicycle that can be used to elicit a work output.

Biomechanics The study of the machine-like aspects of the structure and activity of living organisms, especially humans. It applies the laws of mechanics (a branch of physics) using the procedures of mechanical engineering. It deals with such things as leverage, forces and their effects, velocity, acceleration, momentum, inertia, impulse, and mechanical power and energy.

Bipedal Having only two feet.

Cadence Measured movement or rhythm in walking or running.

Caloric density The amount of energy available in a food, based on its weight.

Calories A measure of energy. The amount of heat needed to change the temperature of 1 kilogram of water from 14.5° C to 15.5° C.

Carbohydrates (CHO) A class of nutrients that supplies energy, serves some structural functions, and contains carbon, hydrogen, and oxygen.

Cardiac output The amount of blood ejected from the ventricles of the heart during a given period of time, usually one minute.

Cardiologist A medical doctor who specializes in the treatment of diseases of the heart.

Cardiovascular Pertaining to the heart, blood, and blood vessels.

Cartilage A type of dense connective tissue consisting of cells embedded in a ground substance or matrix.

Catabolization The metabolic processes by which substances are broken down in the body.

Cellular energetics The molecular mechanisms by which living cells transform fuel into energy for their various needs.

Chondromalacia A condition whereby the cartilage on the inside of the patella erodes, causing a great deal of pain, especially during running.

Cinematography Taking motion pictures, generally with 8 or 16 mm cameras.

Coronary collateral An increase in blood vessels (arteries and arterioles) supplying the heart.

Cytochrome system Iron containing substances found in the mitochondria and important in energy production.

Dehydration A substantial reduction in total body water.

Diaphragm The major muscle of respiration, located at a level with the sixth rib, in front.

Digestion The process by which food is broken down, mechanically and chemically, in the gastrointestinal tract and is converted into absorbable form.

Diuretic A substance that causes an increased loss of water through the kidneys and thus increases urine volume.

Dorsiflexor of foot A muscle located in the front of the lower leg that lifts the toes and front of the foot.

Duck walk A somewhat abnormal walking pattern where the toes are pointed at about a 45° angle away from the direction of movement.

Dynamic Energy, or physical force in motion.

Dysfunction An absence of complete normal functioning.

Dyspnea Labored or difficult breathing usually accompanied by pain or discomfort.

Electrocardiogram (EKG) A record of the electrical activity of the heart.

Electrolyte A solution that conducts electricity. In the human body, electrolytes serve several functions in both blood and tissues.

Endorphin A polypeptide (protein) hormone having opiate-like (inducing sleep or analgesic) qualities and found in the central nervous system.

Endurance-type Long duration exercise, lasting at least 10 minutes and generally performed at less than maximal intensity.

Estrogen A hormone produced by the ovarian follicle and other structures; the female sex hormone.

Fats (lipids) Used for energy. A group of substances that are insoluble in water and soluble in substances such as ether and chloroform. Made of carbon, hydrogen, and oxygen.

Fiber Food substances (carbohydrates) that are not hydrolyzed by acid or alkali.

Force platform A device, usually built into the floor, used to measure force generated between the foot and the ground by an individual during walking, running, or jumping.

Gait A way of moving on foot; a particular fashion of walking or running.

Gastrocnemius One of the two muscles (soleus is the other) that comprise the large calf muscle. Important for the foot push-off phase in running.

Gastrointestinal tract The system made up of the mouth, esophagus, stomach, small and large intestine, and rectum. Digestion takes place here.

Glycogen The storage form of CHO in muscle and liver.

Glycolysis The enzymatic process of breaking down glucose to pyruvate or lactate.

Heat prostration (exhaustion) Results from a serious disturbance of blood flow, similar to shock. Sweating occurs profusely.

Heat stroke A serious condition resulting from a failure of the heat-regulating mechanism of the body. Body temperature may rise to 105–110° F but there is no sweating.

Hemoglobin A substance found in the red blood cell that combines with and carries oxygen in the blood.

High density lipoprotein (HDL) A combination of fat and protein containing 50 percent protein, 25 percent phospholipid, 20 percent cholesterol, and 5 percent triglyceride. Associated with lower risk of heart disease.

High intensity An exercise level that is very close to the individual's maximal capacity.

Homeotherm An organism that is capable of maintaining a relatively constant internal or core temperature.

Homogenous A very similar group of individuals, i.e., of the same relative fitness level.

Hydrostatic weighing A technique whereby the body density is determined from the Archimedes principle (Density = mass ÷ volume). The individual is immersed in water and the volume of his or her body is determined. Body fat is then calculated from prediction formulas.

Hypertension High blood pressure.

Hyperthermia An increase (5–6° F) in internal or core temperature.

Hypothermia A large decrease (5–10° F) in internal or core temperature.

Hypotonic A solution of lower osmotic (less solute) pressure than another. Generally used in reference to plasma.

Intercostal muscles Outer layer of muscles located between the ribs. They are accessory respiratory muscles.

Ischemic Lack of blood to a specific area.

"Junk" foods Foods that contain calories but no protein, vitamins, minerals, or other essential nutrients.

Krebs cycle An aerobic, catabolic pathway by which metabolites of all of the energy nutrients can be processed to make ATP available.

Lactic acid A three-carbon acid that is produced anaerobically from pyruvic acid in muscles.

Lean body weight (LBW) The fat-free weight of the body which includes the muscle mass and various organs and tissues.

Linoleic acid A polyunsaturated fatty acid that is an essential nutrient.

Lordosis Abnormal curvature of the lumbar (lower) spine.

Marathon A road race covering 26 miles, 385 yards.

Medial aspect Refers anatomically to the part of the structure (e.g., foot) that is closest to the center of the body.

Metabolism The sum of all physical and chemical changes that take place within an organism; all energy and material transformations that occur within living cells.

Metatarsal The five long bones in the foot that make up the toes.

Metric mile The more common European mile which covers 1500 meters or 4920 feet.

Mile The U.S. measured mile which covers 5280 feet.

Mineral Inorganic chemical elements that are required in the diet to support the building of physiological structures and the regulation of vital processes in the body.

Mitochondria Structures in the cell where energy production from CHO and fats takes place.

Ml O_2/kg/min A method of expressing VO_2 max, by dividing the oxygen units by an individual's body weight, in kilograms.

Musculoskeletal Pertaining to the muscular and skeletal systems. Since muscles attach to, and cross over bones, the two systems interact closely.

Myelin sheath A fat-like substance that covers certain nerve fibers.

Nitrogen oxide An air pollutant that comes from motor vehicle emissions and the burning of fossil fuels.

Nonsupport phase A phase during the running cycle where both feet are off the ground simultaneously.

Obesity Characterized by an excessive amount of body fat.

Orthopedic Branch of medical science that deals with treatment of disorders involving locomotor structures of the body, such as the skeleton, joints, and muscles.

Orthotic (shoe) Utilization of a device (e.g., arch support) in a shoe to help straighten or correct a deformity of the foot or lower skeletal system.

Ossification The hardening of bone.

Ozone A form of oxygen in which three atoms of the element combine to form the molecule. A dangerous air pollutant.

Peripheral The outermost part or region within a precise boundary, such as the skin of the body.

Physiological Pertaining to the science of the functions of cells, tissues, and organs of the living organism.

Pigeon-toed A somewhat abnormal walking pattern where the toes are pointed at about a 40° angle inward, or toward each other.

Posterior Located behind a part or toward the rear of a structure.

Potassium A mineral element found in the body. It is the principal cation (positive ion) in intracellular fluid.

Pronation (foot) A deviation in alignment between the foot and ankle whereby the medial aspect of the foot becomes a weight-bearing area.

Protein The class of energy nutrient that contains carbon, hydrogen, oxygen, nitrogen, and sometimes sulfur, and is used primarily for structural and regulatory functions.

Protocol The experimental design or format of the testing procedures.

Quadriceps A group of four large muscles located on the front of the upper leg and crossing two joints, the hip and knee.

Radiant heat Heat or energy transferred to or from the environment to the surface of the body in the form of electromagnetic waves.

Relative humidity The ratio of the amount of water vapor in the air at a specific temperature to the maximum capacity of the air at that temperature.

Resynthesis The combining of separate elements or substances to form a coherent whole.

Scoliosis An abnormal lateral spinal deviation.

Sedentarianism The habit of sitting or taking part in very little exercise.

Serum cholesterol A sterol, widely distributed in animals and tissues, occurring in the yolk of eggs, various oils, etc. Serum level is related to risk of heart disease.

Shinsplint A condition characterized by severe pain and irritation on the anterior (front) aspect of the leg. Usually attributed to an inflammation localized primarily in the tendon of the tibialis posterior or to the interossei between the fibula and tibia.

Side-to-side deflection Movement of the body laterally (side-to-side) that usually occurs, to some degree, during running.

Soleus One of the two muscles (gastrocnemius is the other) that comprise the large calf muscle. Important for the foot push-off phase in running.

Starch A general term designating polysaccharides that contain many units of glucose, such as grains, vegetables, and fruits.

Static Masses or forces at rest or in equilibrium; not moving or progressing.

Stress fracture A bone fracture caused by fatigue, overuse, or anatomical abnormalities in skeletal structure.

Stroke volume The amount of blood expelled by the left ventricle during one heart beat.

Substrate A chemical that is the initial reactant in an enzymatic reaction.

Sulfur oxides An air pollutant produced primarily by combustion of fossil fuels such as coal, petroleum, and natural gas.

Supination (foot) The normal alignment of the foot and ankle in running, whereby the lateral border of the foot (bottom) becomes the weight-bearing structure.

Symmetry Exact correspondence of form and constituent configuration on opposite sides of a dividing line or plane or about a center or axis.

Tendonitis Inflammation of a tendon.

Testosterone An androgenic hormone considered to be the principal testicular hormone produced in males.

Therapeutic Pertaining to the application of remedies and the treatment of disease.

Traumatic Caused by or relating to an injury.

Treadmill A motorized device whereby an individual walks or runs on a moving belt at various speeds or elevations.

Vapor The gaseous state of any substance that is liquid or solid under ordinary conditions.

Ventilation The inspiration and expiration of air from the lungs.

Vertical deflection Movement of the body in an upward direction, from the reference point of the ground, during running.

Vitamins The chemical substances that are required in the diet to support growth, maintenance, and well-being. Not used for energy.

VO_2 max (maximal oxygen consumption) The maximum amount of oxygen the body can consume in a given period of time. It is determined primarily by the amount of blood (cardiac output) circulated to the exercising tissues.

"Windchill" factor Defined as that part of the total cooling that is due primarily to the wind action. It is used exclusively in relation to cool or cold environments. Used in expressing the relative discomfort of cold in relation to the absolute temperature and the wind velocity.

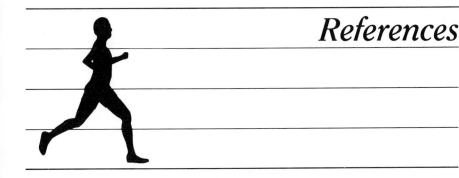

References

Adner, M. M., and Castelli, W. P. "Elevated High Density Lipoprotein Levels in Marathon Runners." *Journal of the American Medical Association* 243(1980): 534–536.

Astrand, I., Guharay, A., and Wahran, J. "Circulatory Responses to Arm Exercise with Different Arm Positions." *J. Appl. Physiol.* 25(1965): 528–532.

Barnard, R. J., Gardner, G. W., Diaco, N. V., Macalpin, R. N., and Kattus, A. A. "Cardiovascular Response to Sudden Strenuous Exercise—Heart Rate, Blood Pressure and Electrocardiogram." *J. Appl. Physiol.* 34(1973): 833–838.

Bergstrom, J., Ahlborg, B., Ekelund, L. G., and Hultman, E. "Muscle Glycogen and Muscle Electrolytes During Prolonged Physical Exercise." *Acta Physiol. Scand.* 41(1957): 305–330.

Buccola, V. A., and Stone, W. J. "Effects of Jogging and Cycling Programs on Physiological and Personality Variables in Aged Men." *Res. Quarterly* 46(1975): 134–139.

Burke, E. J. "Energy Cost of Running at Three Different Stride Lengths." *New Zealand J. Health, P.E., and Rec.* 9(1976): 96–99.

Buskirk, E. L. "Diet and Athletic Performance." *Postgrad. Med.* 61(1977): 229–236.

Caliendo, M. A. *Nutrition and the World Food Crisis*. New York: Macmillan, 1979.

Cavanagh, P. R. Biomechanics of Running. Presented at the 1980 American College of Sports Medicine Meeting, May 28–30, Las Vegas, Nevada.

Cavanagh, P. R., and LaFortune, M. A. "Ground Reaction Forces in Distance Running." *J. Biomechanics* 13(1980): 397–406.

Christensen, E. H. "Contributions to the Physiology of Severe Muscular Work. I. The Blood Sugar During and After Muscular Work." *Arbeitsphysiol.* 4(1931): 128–153.

Cooper, K. H. *Aerobics*. New York: M. Evans, 1968.

Costill, D. L. "Metabolic Responses During Distance Running." *Journal of the American Medical Association* 28(1972): 251–255.

Costill, D. L., Branam, G., Eddy, D., and Sparks, K. "Determinants of Marathon Running Success." *Arbeitsphysiol.* 18(1971): 249–254.

Costill, D. L., Fink, W. J., and Pollock, M. L. "Muscle Fiber Composition and Enzyme Activities of Elite Distance Runners." *Med. Sci. Sports* 8(1976): 96–100.

Costill, D. L., Thomason, H., and Roberts, E. "Fractional Utilization of the Aerobic Capacity During Distance Running." *Med. Sci. Sports* 5(1973): 248–252.

Davis, J. A., Frank, M. H., Whipp, B. J., and Wasserman, K. "Anaerobic Threshold Alterations Caused by Endurance Training in Middle-Aged Men." *J. Appl. Physiol.* 46(1979): 1039–1046.

Girandola, R. N., Wiswell, R. A., and Bulbulian, R. "Effects of Pangamic Acid (B-15) Ingestion on Metabolic Response to Exercise." *Biochem. Med.* 24(980): 218–222.

Hammer, W. M., and Wilmore, J. H. "An Exploratory Investigation in Personality Measures and Physiological Alterations During a 10-Week Jogging Program." *J. Sports Med.* 13(1973): 238–247.

Hartung, G. H., and Farge, E. J. "Personality and Physiological Traits in Middle Aged Runners and Joggers." *J. Gerontology* 32(1977): 541–548.

Hartung, G. H., Foreyt, R. E., Mitchell, R. E., Vlasek, I., and Gotto, A. M., Jr. "Relationship of Diet to High-Density-Lipoprotein Cholesterol in Middle-Aged Marathon Runners, Joggers, and Inactive Men." *N. Engl. J. Med.* 302(1980): 357–361.

Hermansen, L., Hultman, E., and Saltin, B. "Muscle Glycogen During Prolonged Severe Exercise." *Acta Physiol. Scand.* 71(1967): 129–139.

Hogberg, P. "Length of Stride, Stride Frequency, Flight Period and Maximum Distance Between the Feet During Running with Different Speeds." *Arbeitsphysiol.* 14(1952): 431–436.

Holloszy, J. O. "Biochemical Adaptations to Exercise in Aerobic Metabolism," in *Exercise and Sports Science Reviews*, Vol. 1. New York: Academic Press, 1973, pp. 45–68.

Ivy, J. L., Costill, D. L., Fink, W. J., and Lower, R. W. "Influence of Caffeine and Carbohydrate Feedings on Endurance Performance." *Med. Sci. Sports* 11(1979): 6–11.

Issekutz, B., Jr., Birkhead, N. C., and Rodahl, K. "Effect of Diet on Work Metabolism." *J. Nutrition* 79(1963): 109.

Lawrence, J. D., Bower, R. C., Riehl, W. P., and Smith, U. L. "Effects of Alpha-Tocopherol Acetate on the Swimming Endurance of Trained Swimmers." *Am. J. Clin. Nutr.* 28(1975): 205–208.

Pollock, M. L. "Characteristics of Elite Class Distance Runners." *Ann. N.Y. Acad. Sci.* 301(1977): 278–282.

Stein, L., and Belluzzi, J. D. "Brain Endorphins and the Sense of Well-Being: A Psychobiological Hypothesis." *Adv. Biochemical Psychopharmacol.* 18(1978): 299–311.

Vaughan, C. L. "Biomechanics of Running Gait," from *Critical Reviews in Biomedical Engineering*, Vol. 12, 1984.

U.S. Senate Select Committee on Nutrition and Human Needs. *Dietary Goals for the United States*. Washington D.C.: U.S. Government Printing Office, 1977.

Watt, T., Romet, T. T., McFarlane, I., McGuey, D., Allen, C., and Goode, R. C. "Letter: Vitamin E and Oxygen Consumption." *Lancet* 2(1974): 354–35.

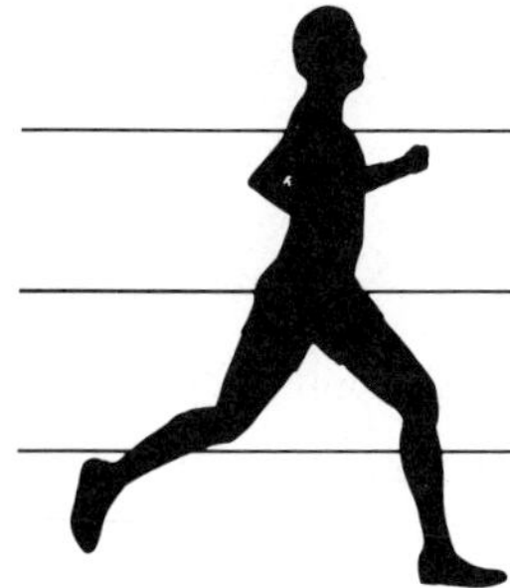

Selected Readings

Textbooks

Astrand, P. O., and Rodahl, K. *Textbook of Work Physiology*. New York: McGraw-Hill, 1985.

Costill, D. L. *Inside Running*. Indianapolis IN: Benchmark Press, 1986.

Daniels, J., Fitts, R., and Sheehan, G. *Conditioning for Distance Running*. New York: John Wiley & Sons, 1978.

Dominguez, R. H. *The Complete Book of Sports Medicine*. New York: Charles Scribner & Sons, 1980.

Fisher, A. G., and Allsen, P. E. *Jogging*. Dubuque IA: Wm. C. Brown, 1980.

Fixx, J. F. *Jim Fixx's Second Book of Running*. New York: Random House, 1980.

Hay, J. G. *The Biomechanics of Sports Techniques*. Englewood Cliffs N.J.: Prentice-Hall, 1973.

Konishi, F. *Exercise Equivalents of Foods*. Carbondale IL: Southern Illinois University Press, 1974.

Mangi, R., Jokl, P. and Dayton, W. *The Runner's Complete Medical Guide*. New York: Summit Books, 1980.

O'Donoghue, D. H. *Treatment of Injuries to Athletes*. Philadelphia: W. B. Saunders, 1976.

Reed, P. B. *Nutrition: An Applied Science*. St. Paul MN: West Publishing, 1980.

Suinn, R. M. *Psychology in Sports*. Minneapolis MN: Burgess Publishing, 1980.

Journals and Magazines

Medicine and Science in Sports and Exercise. American College of Sports Medicine, P.O. Box 1440, Indianapolis IN 46206.

Runner's World. Rodale Press Inc., Emmaus PA 18049.

Running. P.O. Box 350, Salem OR 97308.

The Physician and Sportsmedicine. 4530 W. 77th St., Minneapolis MN 55435.

The Racer's Edge. The Institute for Science and Sport, Box 321, Lake Orion MI 48035.

The Runner. P.O. Box 2730, Boulder CO 80322.

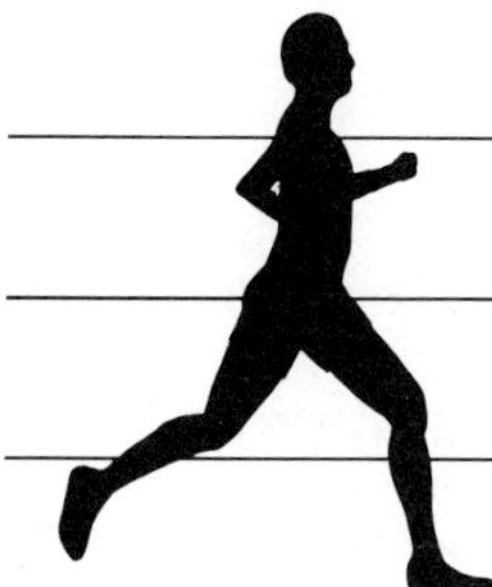

Index

Aerobics, 1
Aerobic system, 7–9, 10
Age
  children, 27, 95, 96–97
  older adults, 39–40, 95, 96–97, 104, 109
Anaerobic cycle, 7, 9, 10, 19
Aouita, Said, 5
Asthma, 17, 98
Athlete's foot, 71
ATP (adenosine triphosphate), 7–8

Bannister, Roger, 5
Biomechanics, 45, 68
Body fat, 2, 13, 22, 37, 79–81

Calories, 2, 75–78, 82, 84–85, 93
Cardiovascular system
  adjustment to exercise, 12
  atherosclerosis, 12
  cardiac output, 11–12
  check-up, 82
  circulation, 13
  disease, 2, 13
  functioning, 24
  heart attack, 12

Cardiovascular system (*Contd.*)
  and hypertension, 13
  pulse rate, 15, 113
Cholesterol, high serum and cardiovascular disease, 13
Cooper, Dr. Kenneth, 3, 5
Cram, Steve, 5

Diabetes, and cardiovascular disease, 13

Equipment
  clothing, general, 29, 34–35, 94–95, 97
  digital chronograph, 35
  shoes, 3, 29–34, 48–52, 57–58, 66–69
  socks, 34, 97
  weights, hand-carried, 60
Exercises
  warm-down, 104–105
  warm-up, 103–105

Fixx, Jim, 12

HDL (high density lipoproteins), 13
"Hitting the wall," 38
Hypertension, and cardiovascular disease, 13

Injuries
- blisters, 63, 70
- connective tissue, 38
- hamstrings, 41, 108–109
- heat-related, 95–98
- knee, 21, 58, 63–64, 68
- musculoskeletal, 37–41
- shinsplints, 58, 64, 67–68
- spinal deviations, 69–70
- stress fractures, 63–64
- tendonitis, 63, 65–66, 73, 103, 106

Kazankina, Tatyana, 5
Kristiansen, Ingrid, 5

Lopes, Carlos, 4, 27

Marathons
- Australia, 3, 95
- Boston, 3, 39
- first women's, 27
- length of, 4
- Los Angeles, 96, 99
- New York, 3, 37, 63
- San Francisco, 3
- training for, 37–38
- world records, 4–5

Menstrual irregularity, 81–82
Mile, American, 5
Mile, metric, 5
Muscles
- biopsy technique, 11
- cells, 7, 38, 40
- fatigue, 7–8
- fibers, 10–11, 18
- injuries, 41
- and stretching exercises, 103–108
- tissue, 8–11
- and ventilation, 16–17

Respiratory system
- described, 16
- dyspnea, 38
- lung capacity, 17
- maximal oxygen consumption (VO_2 max), 17–19

"Runner's high," 25–26
Ryan, Jim, 5

Slaney, Mary, 5
Smoking
- and cardiovascular disease, 13
- and lung capacity, 17

Stress, and cardiovascular disease, 13
Stride, 52–53

Training
- *Fartlek*, 37
- load, 67
- marathon, 37–38
- and the novice, 36, 48, 97
- and older adults, 39–40

Walker, John, 5